HEALTH
FROM THE SEAS
FREEDOM FROM DISEASE

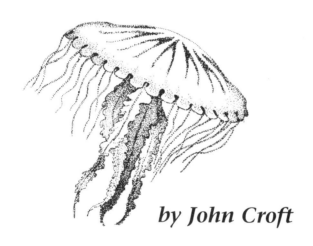

by John Croft

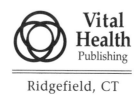

Vital
Health
Publishing

Ridgefield, CT

Health from the Seas: *Freedom from Disease*

Copyright © 2003, John E. Croft

Book Design: interior, Cathy Lombardi; cover, David Richard

Published by: Vital Health Publishing
P.O. Box 152
Ridgefield, CT 06877
Website: www.vitalhealth.net
E-mail: info@vitalhealth.net
Phone: 203-894-1882
Orders: 1-877-VIT-BOOK

Printed in the United States of America
ISBN: 1-890612-29-4

TABLE OF CONTENTS

ACKNOWLEDGMENTS

I am deeply indebted to Dr. Tom Miller, Dr. Douglas Ormrod, Professor Patricia Bergquist, Dr. Paul Davis, and Dr. George Slim for expert scientific guidance through areas of personal weakness. I also extend my thanks to Bruce Russell and Jan Richardson for constantly rescuing me with their skillful manipulation of a computer with a will of its own, and to Healtheries of New Zealand Ltd. for permission to use scientific and clinical data established during my research and development work for their products.

FOREWORD

I feel privileged to have the opportunity to write this book. Almost everyone has a family member, friend, or acquaintance who suffers from one of the diseases for which the natural therapies from the oceans, described in the book, provide an effective treatment. My work as a marine scientist has not provided me with medical training, and I make no pretense to have such skills. All the clinical and medical laboratory work forming the main subject matter of this book has been carried out by specialists in those particular areas of medicine. My privilege has been to be a small part of the overall team of people involved and, perhaps even more, to be the voice for the team.

My whole life has been involved with, and strongly influenced by, the sea: from my birth into a family of seafaring sea captains and fishermen, through my childhood in a small village surrounded on two sides by the sea, to a career and employment involving work on, in, and under the sea!

As a sailor I have witnessed the sea in all its moods—from calm and peaceful to stormy and dangerous—in experiencing its magnitude and enormous power, I have realized the insignificance of our individual human importance, power, or wealth by comparison.

As a diver I have had the benefit of witnessing the enormous wealth of life beneath the surface of both tropical and temperate seas. The biology of the undersea world is one of the most amazing and complex features of our planet, and it is not surprising that it has the potential to provide the treatment for almost all known diseases.

As a marine scientist I have had the honor of researching natural therapeutic products, derived from a variety of marine sources, that have proved to be effective and safe treatments for some of our most debilitating diseases.

I believe that some of the stories in this book relate to the first time in recorded history that the sea has been actively farmed specifically to produce products for use in the treatment of disease. I hope that they produce as much interest for the reader as they have for me.

J. E. Croft, L.R.S.C., M.R.S.N.Z., F.R.S.H.

1

THE SEAS

When we consider that some 70 percent of the surface of our world is covered by water in which some 80 percent of its biological productivity occurs, it should not surprise us to learn that we have, in these waters, a tremendous resource of nutritional and medicinal substances. We have known since very early times that seawater has therapeutic properties and that eating some of the plants and animals it sustains can help to cure certain diseases. We have also known about the tremendous potency of natural toxins in marine creatures such as the pufferfish, the stonefish, and the cone snail. Tetrodotoxin, the poison found in the pufferfish, has no antidote and is several times more potent than morphine. Fortunately, in diluted form its properties are now being used beneficially for relieving pain in terminal cancer patients and also can be applied in epilepsy as an antispasm treatment. However, only during the last four decades has scientific research seriously begun to investigate the potential of new medicinal substances in the seas and oceans.

It may be interesting to note that there is sufficient seawater on our planet to completely submerge all the land masses and that without its presence our existence would not be possible. The seas regulate the earth's atmosphere, controlling the necessary exchange of gases. They also control the temperature and provide the source from which our drinking water is derived by evaporation followed by condensation as rain. In addition to making it possible for our foods to be grown on land by providing the essential moisture and atmospheric conditions, the seas also supply us with some of the most nutritionally valuable foods in the form of fish, shellfish, and seaweeds. To a certain extent, the marine environment also regulates the level of living organisms it contains by a natural and mutually beneficial process for its living occupants. Many of its species produce millions of eggs each time they reproduce, but only a very small proportion of these eggs will develop into young members of the species. The very large number of eggs produced is a means of ensuring that a few will survive to maintain the species because there is no means of protecting the eggs once released. However, those which do not survive are not wasted as they form a part of the food chain for other species. The planktonic broth in the seas must represent the most intense and varied mass of living organisms found on our planet.

There is good reason why products of the sea should be helpful to us both nutritionally and medicinally. The composition of the seas and oceans, where not influenced by freshwater runoff or pollution, is a reasonably consistent solution of mineral salts. Other substances such as proteins and carbohydrates, derived from biological organisms, are also present, but these will vary in their concentration depending on the amount of biological life-forms present. In one cubic meter of seawater there are literally millions of living organisms, ranging from microscopic plants to large fish. To support such an abundance of life calls for a totally balanced environment, and only the seas can provide this. On land this balance does not exist since environmental conditions such as temperature and rainfall can change rapidly and dramatically—a situation that does not occur in the oceans.

Seawater is a natural antibiotic and is an excellent treatment for burns, wounds, and sores. The healing of cuts or sores is noticeably faster if the affected part is regularly immersed in clean seawater. The fact that all the components are naturally dissolved at a balanced level (i.e., there are no excesses such as those which often occur in synthetically made solutions) is almost certainly the reason for the therapeutic benefits attributable to pure seawater.

The Basic Mineral Composition of Seawater

Mineral Ion	Amount Present (parts per million)	Mineral Ion	Amount Present (parts per million)
Chloride	19000	Rubidium	0.2
Sodium	10500	Lithium	0.1
Magnesium	1300	Phosphorus	0.1
Sulphur	900	Barium	0.05
Calcium	400	Iodide	0.05
Potassium	380	Arsenic	0.02
Bromide	65	Iron	0.02
Carbon	28	Copper	0.005
Strontium	13	Zinc	0.005
Boron	4.5	Lead	0.004
Silicon	4.0	Uranium	0.003
Fluoride	1.4	Vanadium	0.0003
Aluminum	0.5	Gold	0.000001

Note: These are values for the open ocean waters; there can be significant variations and also additional elements in different geographical regions. For example, in regions where volcanic activity takes place there can be a significant level of elemental mercury and cadmium present.

Therapeutic Life-Forms from the Sea

With the wealth of life present in the seas, it is certain that some of the life forms will contain substances capable of treating diseases for which a successful synthetic remedy has not yet been established. This is stated with confidence because researchers have already discovered that certain marine sponges contain substances that promise an effective treatment for some forms of cancer. In fact, it appears that the sponges may well provide one of the richest sources of pharmacologically active substances to be found in the sea. The National Cancer Institute in the United

States has been quoted—in my opinion quite appropriately—as predicting that 65 percent of all cancer drugs will have their origin in marine animals and plants. Just a few examples of the compounds derived from marine sponges that are undergoing screening for use in cancer treatment are: Laulimalide from the Okinawan sponge *Fasciospongia rimosa*, Halichondrin B from the New Zealand sponge *Halichondria okadaii*, and Crambescidin from the Mediterranean sponge *Crambe crambe*. There are many, many more from all the oceans of the planet. Some anticancer compounds have even been found in bacteria that inhabit marine animals rather than in the animals themselves. An example is the compound Bryostatin 1, which is derived from a bacteria inhabiting the marine invertebrate *Bugula neritina* (a bryozoan that looks rather like a seaweed but is, in fact, an animal).

While the abundance of algae and animals has yet to be investigated, we can realistically expect to discover new and unique molecular structures that will provide effective and safe treatments for more of our serious diseases.

One of the reasons marine animals and plants contain such highly potent substances—and in many cases novel molecular structures—is the nature of their environment and the influence this has on their ability to grow and survive. Take animals such as sea anemones, for example; they are unable to pursue their food source since they are firmly attached to the seabed. To obtain food, they eject a powerful substance into the water that paralyzes their prey as it swims past. Once the prey is paralyzed, they are then able to secrete powerful digestive enzymes in order to eat it since they do not have the benefit of a mouth with dentures. Starfish and other related marine animals utilize similar digestive processes in order to feed and develop. Imagine the potency of these substances that are able to function with such efficiency in cold saltwater.

Not only do these animals use these potent substances to obtain food for their growth, but they actually create others that they are able to use for protection from predators. The chemical makeup of these substances is of great interest to scientists because they are so potent and, in some cases, highly specific in their action. For medicinal purposes, a product that is very specific to one particular function can be immensely valuable. Often we find that, while a medicinal product has done the job for which we needed it, it has also caused other effects that were not intended. Substances that are able to create just the effect we require and nothing more are highly desirable, and more of such substances are likely to come from the sea.

Because some of the new therapeutic substances being discovered in marine plants and animals have complex and unique molecular structures, it is not unusual to find that we are not able to produce these substances synthetically. This may be because there would be so many stages of synthesis required that the operation would be uneconomic to carry out, or simply that it is beyond our current level of technology. Therefore, in order to ensure that there is a reliable source of the substance available, it is necessary to cultivate the relevant plant or animal by marine farming and to have an appropriate extraction process for obtaining the substance from the organism *in a form that retains its therapeutic activity.*

By coincidence, the need to cultivate certain species of algae and animals by marine farming has helped to curtail the pollution of our coastal waters. It is in the coastal waters that marine farming has to take place for several reasons. Not the least of these is that the natural habitat of the species is normally in the relatively shallow and highly productive waters of the coastal regions. Marine farms also need to be in reasonably sheltered locations with ease of access for operational staff. However, it is into the coastal waters that we tend to discharge our unwanted wastes and, in the past, it has not been uncommon for the financial aspects associated with a waste disposal scheme to counter the aesthetic or recreational values of a particular piece of coastline. Where the coastal region involved is used for marine farming activities, there is a much stronger argument to be presented against the discharge of any such wastes.

If financial fuel needs to be added to this argument, it is useful to point out that productivity, in terms of weight produced per acre, can be at least four to five times higher for marine farms than it is for land farms! There have been instances where it has been possible to utilize what would normally be a polluting discharge to the benefit of fish farming. This occurs where the polluting discharge is hot seawater, previously used for industrial cooling purposes, that can be used subsequently to enhance the growth rate of some fish and also allow the farming of them in areas where the ambient water temperature might otherwise be too cold.

In most cases, however, the argument against the discharge of wastes into the seas needs to be supported by more than aesthetic or recreational components. The combination of the environmental and commercial benefits of marine farming (sometimes referred to as mariculture or aquaculture) can provide this support. This has to be a progressive step toward maintaining what is, after all, the lifeblood of our planet Earth in a survivable condition.

The reader will notice that extracts from the same animals or plants appear in the list of treatments for a variety of different diseases. This is because there are common symptoms to a range of diseases, and the treatment of these symptoms is an important part of the overall management of the disease.

2

ALCOHOL
DAMAGE

In common with many other things in life, consumption of alcohol in moderation need not cause damage to the body. The important word here is *moderation*. However, when consumed in large quantities on a regular basis or, worse still, to excess, alcohol significantly damages a number of vital bodily functions. Those who have occasionally indulged in a reasonably high level of alcohol consumption will have experienced the resultant stomach discomfort, bad taste, and headache generally referred to as a hangover. These symptoms are the result of the alcohol being converted to acetaldehyde in the liver. *Acetaldehyde* is a very toxic substance and, unless it can be broken down quickly to acetic acid and then to carbon dioxide and water, it damages the body in several ways.

To break down acetaldehyde, the liver produces an enzyme called *aldehyde dehydrogenase*. However, under excess alcohol stress, the liver becomes overloaded, resulting in insufficient aldehyde dehydrogenase being produced to deal with the acetaldehyde.

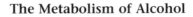

Alcohol

Alcohol Dehydrogenase   ↓

Acetaldehyde

Aldehyde Dehydrogenase   ↓

Acetic acid

↓

Carbon Dioxide   ←   →   Water

Acetaldehyde and some of the by-products of its breakdown to acetic acid cause damage to the liver, brain, and circulatory system. Lowered resistance to disease is another manifestation of excessive acetaldehyde levels. Although the damage caused to the liver and brain cells is possibly the most obvious adverse effect, there are many other, less obvious, deleterious effects such as vitamin and mineral depletion, sexual dysfunction, depression, and hypoglycemia. In particular, the very important B-group vitamins and the minerals calcium, magnesium, and zinc are depleted by heavy alcohol consumption, exacerbating these and other conditions—osteoporosis for instance.

Avoidance of these unpleasant symptoms is, of course, possible by abstinence from alcohol consumption. However, it is possible to consume alcohol in moderation and still avoid or minimize all of the adverse effects described above. Moderation is a nonspecific statement, so a moderate level of alcohol consumption will be quite different for a slightly built female as opposed to a heavily built male. In either case, the level at which the effects of alcohol consumption begin to influence brain cells can usually be recognized by an initial feeling of euphoria, personality change, lessening of depression, and so on.

To minimize the adverse effects of alcohol consumption without having to resort to abstinence, it is necessary to provide the body with the materials it needs to combat these negative effects. It is also necessary to know that these materials are in a suitable form and quantity for the body to assimilate and use at the appropriate sites. It is in this respect that products of the sea are so valuable since they are derived from an environment (seawater) with a remarkable similarity in composition to that of our human body fluids.

On the basis that prevention is better than cure, a prophylactic composition providing antialcohol-damage components (in a convenient capsule form that can be taken prior to alcohol consumption) would seem to be a desirable means of minimizing both the unpleasant hangover feeling and the underlying destruction of the body's cells. Fortunately, the seas provide us with the materials from which just such a natural prophylactic product can be produced.

Minimizing Alcohol Damage: Help from the Sea

The goal of curtailing damage from alcohol consumption can be achieved by employing a nutrient formulation of *multiple* manufactured ingredients. However, the sea provides us with the necessary ingredients in just *two* of its natural products. The principal ingredients required are provided in an extract derived from the cultivated oyster, complemented by the ingredients of a marine alga.

The oyster extract is a natural source of the amino acid taurine. *Taurine* is a very important amino acid because, among its many other health-stimulating functions, it activates the enzyme aldehyde dehydrogenase. This is the enzyme responsible for breaking down the toxic acetaldehyde that results from the oxidation of consumed alcohol. Provided sufficient aldehyde dehydrogenase is available, and active, it will break down all of the acetaldehyde to acetic acid and then to harmless carbon dioxide and water. As mentioned earlier, the toxicity of residual acetaldehyde results in a number of damaging effects on the body.

Other functions of taurine are enhancement of our cellular defense mechanisms and inhibition of liver peroxidation, a very important function for maintaining the health of the liver. Liver peroxidation is the term used to describe the oxidative decomposition of the fatty acids in the liver by reactive oxygen, or free radicals. It can result in chronic liver damage, possibly causing fibrosis of the liver. Also, taurine facilitates our digestion of fat-soluble vitamins and is the second most abundant amino acid in the human brain.

A recent study found that orally administered taurine completely inhibited alcohol-induced hypertension (high blood pressure) in rats (Harada et al.). It may be argued that this study only investigated the effect in rats; however, the fact that the study was concerned with blood pressure, a subject that has been extensively researched in the rat in relation to the human cardiovascular system, makes it reasonable to relate the findings to humans.

Alcohol consumption enhances the loss of minerals from the body, in particular, magnesium and zinc, both of which are important for a healthy metabolism. In addition to its function of reducing the toxic effects of acetaldehyde, taurine also enhances the assimilation of minerals by the body. This is another area where the benefits associated with marine natural products, including oysters, become apparent, because they are naturally rich in all the essential minerals. More importantly, the minerals are present at a level at which the body readily assimilates them because they originate in seawater dissolved at a balanced level. As with all nutrients, it is the amount that we assimilate, not necessarily the amount we consume, that is important.

Taurine is also an essential component of bile and the brain. Brain cell impairment and depression result from excessive alcohol consumption in several ways. In cases of excessive alcohol consumption, vitamin depletion—in particular deficiency of the B-group vitamins—is the cause of neurotransmitter failure and is a characteristic of several other disease states. With respect to brain disorders, research has indicated that a reduced concentration of vitamin B12 (and, incidentally, taurine) is a significant factor in Alzheimer's disease (Mitchell, T.; Csernansky et al.).

A mineral that is very important where alcohol consumption is involved is zinc. Unfortunately, when alcohol is consumed, it is excreted in the urine more rapidly. However, oyster extract contains a healthy level of zinc that functions to synergistically enhance the activity of its natural taurine content.

One other important mineral that is lost more rapidly when alcohol is consumed, is magnesium. Unfortunately, a magnesium deficiency leads to headaches, one of the aftereffects (hangover!) of heavy alcohol consumption. The combined natural mineral content of the oyster extract and algae provide a healthy level of magnesium to counter this loss.

Although the adverse effects of frequent, excessive alcohol consumption will not be reversed by the amount of taurine, minerals, and vitamins naturally present in a few capsules of a formulation containing the components referred to here, the unpleasant "morning after" or "hangover" syndrome that can follow even a moderate drinking session will be minimized. More important, however, will be the reduction in damage caused to the liver and brain cells by vitamin and mineral depletion and the long-term effects of this on the body.

A product from New Zealand that combines an extract derived from the Pacific oyster, and an extract from a marine alga with vitamin B12 and magnesium in a capsule has received wide acclaim for its ability to completely eliminate the "morning after" feeling that follows a drinking session. For those people who suffer hangover effects, even if they have only enjoyed a few social drinks with a meal, this product from the seas, in addition to providing relief and a clear head, performs the more important function of minimizing the more subtle adverse effects on the liver and brain cells.

3

ARTHRITIS

Under the general heading of arthritis, there are many painful and sometimes debilitating disorders. Some of these are classified as degenerative joint disease, or osteoarthritis, while most of the others come under the rheumatoid forms of the disease. In a book such as this, it is neither possible nor justifiable to present a comprehensive coverage of the numerous forms of arthritic disorders. However, a brief description of some of the symptoms associated with the more commonly experienced forms might be helpful.

Osteoarthritis

Degenerative joint disease, or *osteoarthritis*, tends to be a disorder of the elderly, although it will also be a problem for athletes and sports people who experience consistent jarring of the joints over a period of time. Constant heavy loading, such as occurs in the hip joints of people suffering from obesity, will also lead to this condition. In simple terms, osteoarthritis is a condition in which destruction of the cartilage forming the shock-absorbing and spacing of the bones in our joints has occurred. The result of this is that the bone surfaces, which provide the mobility and flexibility in the joint, are in direct contact. Eventually, with constant movement, the smooth surfaces are worn away.

It should not be difficult to imagine the pain and discomfort caused by two roughened bone surfaces grinding together every time the joint is used. These are the main symptoms experienced by sufferers of osteoarthritis, but they are not merely the direct result of the physical factors. Aggravation of the joint caused by the lack of adequate shock absorption and lubrication can create an inflammatory response with related heat and swelling. Another manifestation of osteoarthritis, when it is present in the fingers or toes, is the presence of knobby lumps or spurs on the joints. These bony spurs, which are the result of the joint's attempts to heal itself by producing more cartilage that eventually hardens to a bony structure, severely restrict the flexibility of the joint.

We are all potential candidates for some degree of degenerative joint disease due simply to the aging and natural wear-and-tear process. In the young, healthy body there is a constant breakdown of cartilage that is matched by an equal level of regeneration of new cartilage. This process is called *homeostasis* and is controlled by enzymes. As we age there are gradual changes in our articular cartilage that influence its composition as well as that of the lubricating fluids in the joint space. These changes tend to reduce the flexibility of the cartilage and possibly enhance its vulnerability to enzymic degradation.

However, when degenerative joint disease is not merely a result of the aging process, as in the case of young people or animals, the cause is likely due to the activity of cells called catabolic cytokines that stimulate the production of enzymes responsible for the breakdown of cartilage. This alters the balanced situation (homeostasis) so that the rate of cartilage degradation now exceeds that of regeneration, leading to a breakdown in the joint health.

An important function that can reduce the damaging effect of this process is inhibiting the activity of the catabolic cytokines. If, at the same time, we can stimulate better lubrication and cartilage condition in the joint, we will also relieve the painful symptoms. This is where the products of the sea come in, as we will see later in this chapter.

Some Factors in the Degenerative Processes in Joints

Natural Aging Process	Disease Process
Thinning of articular cartilage with wear	Accelerated rate of articular cartilage degradation
Increasing brittleness and hardening of cartilage	Inflammatory initiation of cartilage damage
Gradual loss of cartilage elasticity	Inflammatory-induced joint fluid swelling
Increased rate of degradation, loss of homeostasis	Abrasion of joint surfaces (chondrocalcinosis)
Viscosity of lubricating fluid reduced	Inflammatory-induced destruction of joint fluid

Rheumatoid Arthritis

This form of arthritis has many different manifestations and can affect all age groups from the young child to the elderly. Unlike osteoarthritis, it is an inflammatory (as opposed to a degenerative) disease. It is a condition that affects the linings of our joints, causing swelling, heat, and pain. In common with osteoarthritis, *rheumatoid arthritis* restricts movement of the joints, but, in this case, it is due to the swelling and inflammation of the lining. Since the pain this induces results in a tendency not to use the affected joint(s), there can also be a wasting of the muscles associated with this disorder.

Rheumatoid arthritis is more prevalent in females than in males, and this would seem to be linked to our hormonal differences. While the specific causes of this disorder are still obscure, several factors and cellular mechanisms that influence the course and severity of the disease are known. For example, immunological influences play a large part, and the stimulation as well as the inhibition of our body's immunomodulatory cells are recognized means of affecting some control over the condition. Hormonal influences play a significant role in rheumatoid arthritis, in particular the prostaglandins. Prostaglandins are a class of fatty acids that are involved in a wide range of bodily functions. With respect to arthritis, some prostaglandins are pro-inflammatory and also sensitize the body to pain. Another group of compounds that are pro-inflammatory and produced by the body in a similar way to the prostaglandins is the leukotrienes. Control of the activity of these compounds is one of the means of moderating the course of the disease and, here again, natural products from the sea can help.

There are other forms of rheumatoid arthritis; they have been given a specific name that is more descriptive of the symptoms. A brief summary of the more common of these may be helpful.

Lumbago or Fibrositis

This is almost certainly one of the most common forms of arthritis and one of the most common causes of absence from work. It is a nonspecific back or neck pain, the term *lumbago* being derived from the lumbar region of the lower back where the symptoms are evident. While the precise cause of this condition is not known, it is frequently related to activities such as heavy lifting or straining the neck by having the head in an unusual position for long periods. The symptoms associated with lumbago and fibrositis result from inflammatory conditions in the connective tissues of the back or neck muscles. The usual pain and stiffness generally experienced with rheumatoid arthritis are present, with the added discomfort of occasional muscle spasms. Lumbago may also result from the degeneration of spinal cartilage, leading to a collapsed vertebral disc. In any event, this form of the disease is very painful and debilitating, but unfortunately does not present any physical manifestation. For this reason it has often been regarded as a malingerer's disorder, where proof of something really wrong has been difficult to establish!

Bursitis

There are two *common* forms of bursitis, one affecting the shoulder and the other the knee. In the case of the knee it is often referred to as "housemaid's knee" because it often results from prolonged kneeling. In both cases it is inflammation of the bursae, small sealed sacs that are designed to lubricate the prominent areas where muscles rub against joints. In the case of housemaid's knee it is the pressure on the bursae that leads to inflammation, whereas in bursitis of the shoulder it is inflammation of the bursae lining the tunnel through which the tendons pass that causes the pain.

Tennis Elbow

This is another inflammatory condition caused by repeated strain on the elbow joint that will result from sporting activities involving a lot of elbow flexing. The same situation could develop in other sports such as golf, badminton, and even winding sheet winches on sailing boats. It is also possible to suffer bursitis of the elbow due to inflammation of the bursae through persistent leaning on the elbow. This is quite different from tennis elbow and related to bursitis rather than joint inflammation.

Still's Disease

As mentioned earlier, rheumatoid arthritis can affect people of any age, but when it is present in young children it is known as *Still's disease*. This rare condition tends to affect more girls than boys. Fortunately the disorder is usually temporary, and most young people will grow out of it by their teens. Because it is basically rheumatoid arthritis, it presents the same symptoms already described above.

Ankylosing Spondylitis

This is a condition where inflammation in the joints of the spinal column has created bony growths that have then fused segments together to form a rigid spine. Obviously this is a serious barrier to movement; however, the condition will respond to treatment and, fortunately, is often temporary in nature. This is one instance when males, rather than females, are more likely to encounter the condition.

Influential Factors in Arthritis

There are many opinions with regard to the causes of, and influences on, arthritic diseases. As mentioned earlier, the cause of most of the forms of arthritis are well understood and there are certain features that are common to many of the various forms. Where there are differences of opinion, these are usually more related to the influence of factors such as diet, climate, or environmental circumstances on the course of, rather than the cause of, the disease. A brief discussion on the more frequently expressed opinions may be helpful.

Stress
There can be little doubt that stress is one of the most influential factors affecting the course of the inflammatory arthritic diseases. It has been documented that among women who were pregnant during the Second World War there was a significant increase in the number who suffered from arthritis. This is believed to be a direct result of the stress these women endured— not knowing if their husbands would ever return, carrying a baby during such violent times, and other factors. Whether these stress factors were involved in actually causing the disease is uncertain, but there is a strong possibility that they were influential. It is also known that stress can cause flare-ups and regression in people with arthritis, even though they may be undergoing successful treatment at the time. What is sometimes not fully

appreciated is the number of different ways in which stress can be manifested. Sometimes factors that seem to be associated with a totally unrelated situation make their effect in the form of stress. For example, extremes of cold or heat exhibit the same influence in aggravating inflammatory conditions; this may be due to the fact that both of these situations put the body in a stressful condition. We may regard either as merely a discomfort, but the very fact that we are uncomfortable means that our body is under stress. The same sort of situation can occur if we have to attend a meeting about which we are very nervous. There is no apparent physical change in us but our body is under stress due to the tension and anxiety we have built up about the meeting. When we experience these discomforts or anxiety situations, there are physiological changes taking place which, in very simple terms, alter our body chemistry and can therefore affect other processes taking place, such as inflammatory reactions. There are so many examples of these manifestations of stress that we should easily recognize. The loss of appetite when we are very anxious or nervous, the tendency to perspire when afraid or worried, blushing when embarrassed—all of these involve physiological changes from our normal condition. Getting somewhat more basic, we can even relate our stress experiences to the natural tendency in animals for a "fight-or-flight" response where the adrenal gland starts to pump out adrenaline, the hairs in some parts of the body stand up, and all systems are fully alert. These are simply natural responses to a particular or overly prolonged situation, but certainly create a stressful condition in the body when overstimulated. While this last example is one that would normally be of a very temporary nature, it does illustrate the effect that external influences, quite unrelated to medicine, can have on our body's functions and its stress level.

Ironically, it is not only unpleasant or worrying situations that cause stress. Emotional factors such as excessive excitement or joy can also be stressful in physiological terms. It is more often the unpleasant situations, however, that are responsible for our stress-related problems.

Diet

While it is reasonable to assume that diet will have an influence on our body's physiological activities, it is not certain that it has the effect on arthritic disorders that is often claimed. Some people claim that eating anything acidic, such as fruit, is detrimental to them, while another group will say that red meat is what causes problems for them. There are other examples cited, such as dairy products, sugars, and so on. There will be no doubt in the mind of the person involved that the particular food has the effect of aggravating their condition. Where there may be some doubt is whether it is the direct action of the food concerned that is creating the aggravation or whether it is due to an indirect effect, such as adverse reactions in the digestive processes to this food that lead to discomfort and thus stress. In other words we have a stress-related problem rather than a biochemical problem. In the end, the net result is the same: If a certain food creates problems, then don't use it!

There are certain dietary recommendations that can be offered, which really apply to all conditions. Everyone needs a balanced intake of essential nutrients in order to maintain metabolic functions in good working order. The critical part is in the assimilation of the nutrients from the food we eat. We can only benefit from the proteins, fats, carbohydrates, vitamins, and minerals in our foods if we are able to assimilate them into our systems. As a rather extreme example—but nevertheless indicative of the point being made—if we ate a perfectly balanced diet but all the foods were sealed tightly in plastic when we ate them, we would not assimilate any of the goodness of the diet as it would pass straight through undigested. Thus, we need to eat foods that are easily assimilated into our systems in order to benefit from their nutritive, and sometimes therapeutic, properties.

A balanced diet would include fresh vegetables, seafood, dairy products, fruits, and some meats (particularly liver and kidneys). No doubt there will be certain people who will have allergic reactions to one or another of these items, in which case that item should be left out. The basic principle is to ensure a balance of the things that are essential to our well-being. If we are able to do this, we have a much better chance of preventing diseases and of fighting them should we be unfortunate enough to contract one. One of the advantages that many kinds of seafood offer is the balance of nutritional components they naturally contain—all being derived from the balance of seawater. The *New Zealand green-lipped mussel* is an excellent example of this balance, having a rich protein, carbohydrate, and mineral content plus a healthy level of omega-3 fatty acids and the B-complex vitamins.

Climate
The arthritic diseases are widespread and afflict people living in a broad range of climatic conditions. There is no doubt that climatic circumstances can aggravate arthritic conditions, but it is highly improbable that they are responsible for causing the conditions. People living in the heat of the tropical areas suffer from the disease in similar proportion to those living in the very cold regions of the world. As with the common cold, our resistance to disease can be lowered by exposure to unfavorable climatic conditions. But the causative virus or other factor must be present if we are to contract the disease. Hence, climate as such tends to be an aggravating factor if it creates discomfort due to excessive heat, cold, or humidity. Here we are back to the stress factor again!

On a positive note, it is not difficult to see that living in a pleasant, sunny climate with low humidity and a comfortable temperature range will offer the best chance of comfort and freedom from climatic stress problems.

Treating Arthritis: Help from the Sea

There are several natural and effective treatments for the varied symptoms of arthritis that can be derived from marine sources. However, the most universal and well-researched treatment discovered so far is the New Zealand Green-Lipped Mussel Extract. I have been privileged to have been responsible for the coordination of the scientific and clinical research into the therapeutic properties of this product over the past twenty-seven years. Because there has been such an extensive amount of research carried out on this product, the reporting of the findings, even in condensed form, will form a significant part of this chapter. I make no apology for this because my long experience with the product, with the research scientists, and, in particular, with thousands of sufferers of arthritis worldwide has confirmed my earlier faith that, in the Green-Lipped Mussel Extract, we have a unique, safe, and highly effective natural product of the sea.

Green-Lipped Mussel Extract

The discovery of the beneficial properties of the New Zealand Green-Lipped Mussel Extract came from work done in the United States. In the 1960s, researchers began to seriously study the marine environment in the search for possible treatments for cancer. Large sums of money were available for this particular line of research, and all avenues ripe with the potential for nature to yield a therapy for cancer were being explored.

Out of this research effort came the finding that the New Zealand green-lipped mussel, while not having any beneficial properties for the treatment of cancer, exhibited significant anti-inflammatory activity. Since anti-inflammatory agents are extensively used in the treatment of arthritis, one of the world's most widespread and debilitating diseases, it was obvious that this mussel may have an important role to play as a treatment for arthritis.

Nevertheless, it was necessary to establish that the anti-inflammatory properties of the Green-Lipped Mussel Extract were effective when humans or animals consumed the material orally, as the original indications would only have come from rats. It was also necessary to establish that the material was safe when taken in therapeutic doses, and that it did not have unpleasant or dangerous side effects. It could not be assumed that, simply because this material was extracted from a shellfish eaten extensively as a food, it would be quite safe to use in a concentrated form or would be free of adverse side effects.

In New Zealand, the McFarlane family company, which had pioneered the farming of the green-lipped mussel, provided the mussels for the research in the United States and was the only company cultivating this shellfish at the time. Continuing their pioneering work, they set up McFarlane Laboratories to undertake this essential work and commissioned the necessary research programs at the University of Auckland. This led to the development and production of the Green-Lipped Mussel Extract, which is now used worldwide.

By far the greatest amount of research into the properties of the mussel extract has been carried out by leading scientists in the Department of Medicine at the University of Auckland (Miller et al., Couch et al.). However, additional studies have also been done by some of the major pharmaceutical companies and other independent clinical and laboratory researchers in other countries around the world. The results of all this work, which included an investigation to rule out the possibility of adverse effects on fetal development if taken during pregnancy (*teratogenicity*), demonstrated that the mussel extract was a safe and effective anti-inflammatory product.

While laboratory and clinical studies are required to prove the effectiveness of a product under controlled conditions, the real experts in arthritic disorders are the people who suffer from them. Very valuable information has come from these people during the past twenty years, indicating just what they were suffering and how the mussel extract had helped them. These reports were completely unsolicited and, in fact, still continue to be received.

Some of these personal reports have been written by medical practitioners because arthritis has no respect for profession. In such cases there has often been very detailed clinical information explaining the recovery process from a medical standpoint, which has been particularly valuable. However, the reports from all arthritis sufferers, detailing their particular story of a gradual and progressive relief from pain and stiffness, have been important as proof of the effectiveness of the product. Many of these reports, although originating in different countries, and coming from a wide variety of age groups, have described almost identical recovery patterns. This information, albeit subjective for each individual case, when considered collectively, becomes valuable, objective clinical evidence for the product's efficacy.

Not all the reports have been about human success; many have related to the renewed quality of life for an aged pet following treatment with the mussel extract prepared in tablet form for dogs or cats. From being pain-ridden and reluctant to move, these pets were described as meeting their returning owners at the door anxious to get out for some exercise!

Other pets have been described as becoming puppy- or kittenlike in their playfulness, despite having been lethargic prior to taking mussel extract.

Even horses have responded to treatment with the mussel extract to such an extent that animals, once considered only suitable for stud purposes due to joint disease, were able to resume racing—and win!

What Does the Mussel Extract Do?

In general, approximately 70 percent of arthritis cases benefit by using the mussel-extract product. The degree of benefit varies from person to person, and this variation is explained in more detail later.

The benefit comes as relief from pain and improvement in general mobility. Usually the improvement in these conditions is gradual and progressive; it is also usually long-lasting and not just temporary. Normally, the first thing to be noticed is a reduction in pain, which is then followed by a gradual improvement in grip strength, freedom of movement or other mobility, dependent on the nature of the original problem.

The assessment of the product, based on clinical trials, presents the changes in the arthritic condition in strictly clinical terms, which is of value to doctors (Gibson et al.; Huskisson et al.; Caughey et al.; Larkin et al.; Orima et al.; Ankenbauer-Perkins et al.; Lambnert et al.; Kendall et al.; Hawkins, T.). However, for the nonmedically trained person, it is usually of more value to hear about the experiences of other sufferers expressed in practical terms.

The experiences of many of the people who have communicated with McFarlane Laboratories fall into a similar pattern. Usually, the first thing they noticed was a gradual reduction in pain. For example, people with hip problems have said that they noticed they were getting a full night's sleep instead of waking in pain whenever they moved in their sleep. This was their first indication that the product was working.

Others have commented that they suddenly noticed they were able to zip up a dress or comb their hair first thing in the morning without the usual pain. People have often said that the initial relief from pain encouraged them to use the affected muscle or joint, leading to a gradual increase in its freedom of movement. This use of the affected part of the body has, in itself, been therapeutic and has led, in many cases, to full recovery of mobility or the ability to grip things. Typical examples of these recoveries have ranged from the person who has simply been able to hold a pen again or take the top off of a jar, to someone who has been able to resume playing the piano or holding work tools again, to major changes where a person has been able to discard a walking stick or even a wheelchair.

Most people, having experienced the benefit of relief from pain and stiffness, will not risk any possibility of a return to their original condition and continue to take a reduced dosage each day whether they need to or not. Where this small daily maintenance dose is necessary, the number of capsules to be taken has been determined by trial and error since it is subject to the individual person's needs.

The mussel-extract product has another, secondary, beneficial effect that almost certainly helps in the recovery process for those taking it specifically for relief from arthritis. This effect has been described in various ways, such as "a desire to be active," "a feeling of well-being," "enhanced vitality." There can be little doubt that experiencing such an effect is likely to enhance the progress of recovery.

Animals Also Benefit

Outside of controlled clinical trials, one of the most positive indications of the effectiveness of a product is its effect on animals. Animals are not subject to the psychological effects of taking medicinal products; therefore, if a product works for an animal, it rules out the possibility of a placebo effect. The mussel-extract product works extremely well for animals, in particular arthritic and old dogs.

The secondary effect of enhancing vitality is also very noticeable in animals. Some racehorses, treated with the extract for leg problems, had to be dope-tested because their form improved so dramatically and so quickly. Fortunately, the product is not a stimulant, and the tests came out negative!

Another interesting feature that has been reported by many pet owners using the mussel extract on a pet is the regrowth of fur and hair where bald patches previously existed.

Typical comments from pet owners who have used the mussel extract on their animals have been, "I could not believe that my old dog could change so dramatically in such a short time, from his lethargic, uninterested state to the vibrant dog that now greets me at the door with his leash in his mouth anxious to get out for a walk." Another comment relates to the fact that the owner no longer has to lift the animal into the car or carry it upstairs. Cat owners have said that their cat, which used to do nothing more energetic than drag itself to its food bowl, now catches birds on the wing. Not so good for the bird lovers, yet perhaps if the birds also took the extract, the cat wouldn't manage to catch them! Although it may sound strange, there have even been reports from some veterinarians that they have used the extract with budgies and parrots because the birds had developed arthritis in their feet and were having difficulty holding onto the perch.

Where horses have been treated with the mussel extract, it has usually been racing animals that have injured a leg or developed a condition known as *splints* through racing on hard ground. Whereas treatment with drug therapy usually meant the horse was put out to pasture for 3 to 6 months during treatment, when the mussel extract was used, they were back racing within about 6 weeks. Not only were they back on the track but in some cases were significantly exceeding their previous racing form.

The daily dosage for animals is based on their body weight at 17 milligrams per kilogram of body weight. For dogs and cats, the product is presented in the form of tablets or specially designed treats the animals find appealing. For horses, it is presented as a powder which is then mixed in with the daily feed.

Owners usually see results in as little as 10 days for dogs and cats (much less than the average time for the human animal).

How Does the Mussel Extract Work?

Because there has been so much excellent research work done on the mussel extract, it is possible to explain why it has such beneficial properties for the treatment of arthritis. There are basically three contributory elements in the extract that combine to make it a powerful, yet safe, treatment.

The main anti-inflammatory component in the extract is a glycogen complex, which can be shown by the standard pharmacological techniques used in the assessment of medicinal products to have a significant effect in suppressing inflammation. There are several ways in which an inflammatory condition can be controlled. It seems that the extract works on at least two of these, as described here. However, these are very much simplified explanations of what are, in fact, complex biochemical processes that take place in our bodies.

In our blood we have cells called *neutrophils* that are some of the soldiers in our defense system. These neutrophils are constantly circulating in the bloodstream with some attaching to the blood-vessel walls and then releasing again so that, at any one time, there may be 50 percent of the neutrophils sticking to the blood-vessel walls and the other 50 percent circulating. If an inflammatory stimulus occurs (as is the case in many types of arthritis), there is a change in the nature of the blood vessels that allows some of those neutrophils that are attached to the walls to escape through the walls and attack the site of the inflammatory stimulus, thus causing inflammation, swelling, and pain.

What some drug products and the mussel extract can do is prevent the neutrophils from escaping and attacking the inflammatory stimulus. This is achieved by either blocking the activation signal, which tells the neutrophils to attack, or by blocking the activation sites so that the neutrophils cannot attach.

This activity does not compromise the body's resistance to infection because the suppression of neutrophil function is moderate. Research (published in the *British Journal of Experimental Pathology* in 1986) has shown that neutrophil function has to be reduced by more than 90 percent before host defenses to infection are compromised (Miller et al.).

Another way in which the mussel extract acts as an anti-inflammatory agent involves substances called *prostaglandins*. Prostaglandins are a group of hormones, naturally present in the body, that are responsible for regulating many of the body's functions. During some of these functions, the pathways can result in inflammatory processes that involve the conversion of arachidonic acid to pro-inflammatory prostaglandins and leukotrienes. There are several steps in these conversion pathways and the blocking of just one of these steps can be sufficient to prevent the formation of the undesirable compounds.

The production of the pro-inflammatory prostaglandins from endogenous arachidonic acid is carried out by enzymes called *cyclo-oxygenases*. However, there are other prostaglandins that the body needs for normal functions and these are also produced by cyclo-oxygenase enzymes. The cyclo-oxygenase enzyme that produces the prostaglandins needed for normal functions is called a *constitutional cyclo-oxygenase* and is known as COX1. The cyclo-oxygenase enzyme responsible for the production of the pro-inflammatory prostaglandins is an induced form known as COX2. One of the major problems associated with the use of nonsteroidal anti-inflammatory drugs for the treatment of arthritis is that they block or inhibit the activity of both COX1 and COX2 enzymes. This results in the protective functions for the stomach lining, aggregation of blood platelets, and other desirable activities of the "good" prostaglandins being destroyed. It is obviously desirable therefore to have a product that will selectively inhibit COX2 activity without affecting the constitutional COX1 activity. Recent research studies at the University of Otago, Wellington School of Medicine, have now established that the Green-Lipped Mussel Extract performs this selectivity in its inhibition of prostaglandin synthesis in the body. While some of the newer, nonsteroidal anti-inflammatory drugs are COX2 *preferential*, the Green-Lipped Mussel Extract goes one better in being COX2 *selective*. It is the long-chain fatty acids naturally present in the extract that perform this important function.

The two anti-inflammatory activities just described make the product a very valuable, perfectly natural treatment for the types of arthritis that have an inflammatory component. Most forms of arthritis do involve an inflammatory component. Even osteoarthritis, which is not an inflammatory condition, usually has associated inflammation caused by the degraded bone surfaces rubbing together.

The mussel extract contains, as part of its natural composition, substances called *mucopolysaccharides* (also known as *glycosaminoglycans*), and these substances are influential in the production and repair of cartilage, synovial fluids, tendons, and skin. Recently there has been a great deal of publicity for two groups of compounds—the chondroitin sulfates and the glucosamines—indicating the benefit that these can give in the treatment of arthritic disorders. We can be pleased therefore to discover that these compounds form part of the mucopolysaccharide content naturally present in the mussel extract.

Glucosamines are sugar molecules. When a number of them are coupled together in the form of a chain, they make mucopolysaccharide molecules. Glucosamine forms the initial building unit for the synthesis of *chondroitin sulfate*, one of the mucopolysaccharides, although it first becomes galactosamine because chondroitin sulfate is made up of a chain of galactosamine molecules. Hyaluromic acid, however, another beneficial mucopolysaccharide, is made up of glucosamine molecules.

If the mucopolysaccharide molecules are then coupled with protein molecules, a new molecule called a *proteoglycan* is formed. The proteoglycans are important space-filling molecules in what is known as the extracellular matrix. Simply expressed, this means that they fill up gaps in the body's structure, such as the spaces around joint cavities. By doing this they act as shock absorbers as well as lubricants for joint surfaces. They are able to achieve this because of the very strong attraction of proteoglycan molecules for water.

Thus, in one natural product—New Zealand Green-Lipped Mussel Extract—we have three very effective treatments for the various forms of arthritis.

To summarize:

- The mussel extract contains a glycogen complex molecule that has significant anti-inflammatory activity. It suppresses inflammation by blocking neutrophil emigration.

- The mussel extract contains long-chain fatty acids that suppress inflammation by blocking the synthesis of prostaglandins and leukotrienes from endogenous arachidonic acid. It is COX2 selective and therefore only blocks the undesirable prostaglandins, allowing the constitutional COX1 prostaglandins to perform their protective functions.

- The mussel extract contains mucopolysaccharides that relieve arthritic symptoms by enhancing joint lubrication, boosting shock resistance, and rebuilding cartilage.

- It was mentioned earlier that there is a secondary, beneficial side effect experienced when the mussel extract is used. This effect is the enhancement of vitality and endurance. There is absolutely no doubt that this effect occurs because it is so often described by people from their own or a pet's experience. It has also been demonstrated in a double-blind clinical trial in which the endurance and performance of athletes using the product was measured against athletes who did not use the product (Lambert et al.). Whether it occurs as a result of one of the mechanisms described above, or simply because the release from pain and increase in mobility becomes the catalyst, is not so important. What is significant is that it happens!

Note: Gout is a form of arthritis that should *not* be treated with the mussel extract. The reason for this is that gout is a disorder in which the body produces an excess of uric acid, and this excess is deposited in the joints in the form of crystals. Unfortunately, along with cheese and wine, shellfish contain a reasonably large amount of a purine nitrogen compound, which is a precursor for uric acid. In other words, by consuming these products we would be providing the fuel for the body to make even more uric acid!

Shark Cartilage

This product came to prominence during the 1980s mainly because it received a significant amount of publicity as a potential treatment for cancer patients. More on this follows in a later chapter. However, shark cartilage had also been shown to be effective for the relief of symptoms in arthritis sufferers. Some of the mechanisms involved in tumor development and metastasis are also involved in rheumatoid arthritis, and it therefore seems reasonable to assume that a treatment that is effective for one disorder might well be beneficial for treating the other.

In addition, shark cartilage is a good source of marine glycosaminoglycans, which we have already heard about in the mussel extract. In fact, shark cartilage generally has a slightly higher content of the glycosaminoglycans than the mussel extract. Whereas the level in mussel extract will range from about 2 to 6 percent, that in good-quality shark cartilage will range from about 4 to 10 percent. Unfortunately, there have been a considerable number of wildly exaggerated claims made for the level of glycosaminoglycans by competitive marketers and, while in many cases analytical documents have been produced to support the claims, it is a simple fact that the use of inappropriate analytical methods can produce totally incorrect results that yield a much higher figure than is actually the case.

The source of shark cartilage also has an influence on the yield and quality of product in terms of its glycosaminoglycan content. For example, product made from some species is superior to that from others, and product made from the fins or gills of the shark is often superior to that made from its cartilaginous backbone. Since shark cartilage is normally produced from sharks caught for use as food (much of the fish used for fish and chips is shark), it is not usually possible to simply select the best species for the production of the cartilage powders.

Shark cartilage is produced in a powder form, followed by encapsulation or tabletting for ease of consumption.

How Does Shark Cartilage Work?

There are two principal activities naturally occurring in shark cartilage. Both can be described as *primarily chondroprotective* with secondary anti-inflammatory functions.

We have already seen how the glycosaminoglycans present in Green-Lipped Mussel Extract provide a chondroprotective function in our joints by combining with water in the joint to produce large lubricating and shock-absorbing molecules. The same glycosaminoglycans are present in shark cartilage and they provide the very same function in the joints. Chondroitin sulfate is by far the most abundant glycosaminoglycan present, comprising about 80 percent of the glycosaminoglycan content. In addition, the glycosaminoglycans serve to inhibit cartilage degradation by inhibiting the activity of the particular enzymes that cause this. These enzymes are called metalloproteinases and elastases and they facilitate the natural breakdown of cartilage. In the healthy joint this is not a problem because regeneration is occurring at about the same rate. However, in the arthritic joint there can be an excess of the destructive enzymes, which creates an unfavorable balance.

Another beneficial function of the glycosaminoglycans is in the absorption of free radicals. In the arthritic joint, damage-causing, oxidative free radicals such as nitric oxide are undesirable, and antioxidant activity (binding these free radicals and preventing their independent functioning) is one of the treatment processes.

The other main activity of shark cartilage is *angiogenesis inhibition*—thought to be due to a protein component called Troponin 1, although other protein components could also be involved (Davis, P. F. et al.; Oikawa, T. et al.). Literally translated, angiogenesis means "the birth of new blood vessels." Although this is normally an essential bodily function, uncontrolled angiogenesis can lead to a variety of health problems. In the case of rheumatoid arthritis, the problem is destruction of joint cartilage caused by abnormal capillary growth. By inhibiting angiogenesis, shark cartilage reduces this cartilage-destructive process.

Are There Any Adverse Side Effects?

- Allergy reactions common to seafood are possible.

- Shark cartilage contains a significant amount of calcium and, if consumed in large amounts over a long period, could possibly lead to the development of kidney stones.

- More of a caution than a side effect is the fact that shark cartilage should not be consumed by anyone who is recovering from invasive surgery, is pregnant, or is undergoing wound healing. In these instances, angiogenesis should not be inhibited.

Note: Shark cartilage products *should not be taken together with fruits or vegetables* (including juices) because they contain bioflavonoids. Bioflavonoids will bind (attach) to proteins and, because the angiogenesis-inhibiting active component in shark cartilage is protein, there is the potential that its inhibiting activity will be lost. Taking the product at least two hours before a meal involving fruits or vegetables and using water or milk as an aid to swallowing the capsules or tablets will avoid this.

Sea Cucumber

The sea cucumber, which is also known as Beche-de-Mer, is a relative of the starfish and sea urchin family of echinoderms. It is widely distributed throughout northern and southern hemisphere waters and has been highly regarded for its therapeutic and culinary properties by the Chinese people for centuries. In the past three decades a significant amount of international research has been conducted on the humble sea cucumber, mainly aimed at identifying the bioactive components responsible for its antifungal and anti-inflammatory properties. Although the species from different areas vary in appearance and size, the illustration in this book is typical of the basic sea cucumber. Viewing this picture makes one wonder if the Chinese people, who regard sea cucumber as a restaurant delicacy, would have quite the same enthusiasm if they saw the animal in its natural form and environment.

Laboratory studies investigating the therapeutic properties of sea cucumber found that preparations of this animal exhibited high anti-inflammatory activity when the product was injected, but only a weak activity when administered orally (Whitehouse, M. W. & Fairlie, D. P.).

Contrary to this, a 6-month, placebo-controlled clinical trial in Australia, in which 34 patients took part, concluded that sea cucumber improved the condition of the 18 rheumatoid arthritis patients receiving the product, whereas the 16 patients on placebo showed no improvement (Hazelton, R. A.).

However, it is not unusual for laboratory studies and clinical studies to produce conflicting results when natural products are being studied.

What Does Sea Cucumber Do?

The outer wall of the sea cucumber is rich in glycosaminoglycans which, as we have seen earlier, have a beneficial effect in treating osteoarthritis. Thus, in common with mussel extract and shark cartilage, sea cucumber will inhibit the degenerative processes taking place in the joints and possibly stimulate regenerative functions. Injected sea cucumber preparations exhibit a significant anti-inflammatory activity in laboratory rats, but only a weak activity when introduced orally. This anti-inflammatory activity has been shown to be the result of the inhibition of neutrophil activity, which is similar to that of the mussel extract. However, the mussel extract also works when orally administered. It is possible that the specific carbohydrates responsible for this bioactivity of sea cucumber are broken down in the digestive system and thus are unable to get to the active sites in the body. Possibly a tablet with a protective coating to prevent early breakdown would overcome this problem.

In addition to these activities, sea cucumber has also been shown to have analgesic properties that would certainly be beneficial for symptomatic relief in arthritic patients (Yaacob, H. B. et al.). Although the research that demonstrated this property of sea cucumber was conducted using mice models, a comparison was made with both aspirin and morphine in the same models. The relative degrees of analgesia induced were such that it is reasonable to assume that they would apply equally to humans.

Are There Any Adverse Side Effects?

• Allergy reactions common to seafood are possible.

• Possible mild nausea due to the nature of the product origin could occur.

There have been no incidences of toxicity associated with the use of sea cucumber for treating arthritic symptoms.

Author's Note: There are a number of companies marketing imitation products containing only green-lipped mussel powder and claiming that its properties are the same as those of the Green-Lipped Mussel Extract powder referred to in this chapter (and the material I have had the privilege of researching for the past 30 years). This has created a considerable amount of confusion. To avoid being misled by imitation products, readers who wish to try the Green-Lipped Mussel Extract powder discussed in this chapter should confirm that the product being offered contains the active ingredient Biolane GLME, or in North America, Glycomarine.

4

ATHEROSCLEROSIS

Atherosclerosis is a form of arterio-sclerosis in which a fatty plaque builds up on the arterial walls. This can be likened to the situation in rivers where the river twists and turns and the sediment builds up on the inside of the bends with the deep water flowing round the outside. In our arteries the deposits of fatty plaque tend to build up on the inside of the bends where the blood flow is slower. Over time the buildup of this plaque leads to constriction of the arterial blood flow and can result in problems such as high blood pressure or angina.

The formation of fatty plaque in our arteries is related to the level of fats, principally cholesterol, being carried around in our blood serum. The term hypercholesterolemia is given to the situation where the level of cholesterol in the serum is excessive, and it is this condition that predisposes a person to the problems of atherosclerosis. It is important to recognize that all cholesterol is not harmful and, in fact, we are very dependent on cholesterol for a healthy existence. However, we come back to the role of *balance*—the key to harmony in every aspect of life! It is the balanced level of fats and, in particular, the balanced ratio of the different forms of fats (called lipids) that is important. We will discuss this aspect further in Chapter 7, which addresses cholesterol problems in general.

Treating Atherosclerosis: Help from the Sea

Atherosclerosis can be treated by drug therapy, commonly by a group of drugs known as *statins*. However, these treatments can be accompanied by unpleasant side effects. A product of the oceans that does not create unpleasant side effects and has been shown in laboratory studies to be effective in inhibiting the formation of atherosclerotic plaque is a welcome addition to the therapies available (Ormrod, D. J. et al.). This product is called *chitosan* and it can be prepared from a variety of marine sources. It can also be produced by a fermentation process involving certain fungi, but, in the author's experience, current supplies are all derived from one or more marine sources.

Chitosan

Chitosan is a polysaccharide (a sugar with more than eight re-peating molecules joined together). It is derived mainly from the shells of lobster, crayfish, shrimps, and crabs. However, in New Zealand, a superior form of chitosan is derived from the backbone of the squid (known as a *squid pen*). The two forms of chitosan are differentiated by the prefix alpha or beta, relating to the form derived from the crustaceans mentioned above or the squid pen, respectively. The reason why beta-chitosan is superior to alpha-chitosan is related to how chitin, which is the building block or main structural component of crustacean shells and squid pens, is changed into chitosan. Squid-pen chitin requires less processing than crustacean chitin and this results in a more active product on a weight-for-weight basis.

The molecules which, linked together, form chitosan are par-tially deacetylated acyl glucosamine molecules, and the alpha and beta forms of these produce the alpha and beta forms of chitosan.

Chitosan is a fascinating substance because it has so many different applications, from wound-healing bandages and waste-treatment processes to influencing cholesterol levels and inhibiting atherosclerosis. In this chapter we are only interested in the application for inhibiting atherosclerosis and the mechanism by which this can be achieved.

In the trial referenced earlier, the administration of a chitosan-supplemented diet resulted in a substantial and highly significant reduction in both blood cholesterol and atherosclerosis. The mechanism for the inhibition of atherosclerosis is thought to be the binding of bile acids by chitosan. Under normal circumstances, bile is secreted by the liver into the intestine, aiding the digestion and absorption of nourishment from foods and solubilizing lipids (fats and oils) ready for excretion. Some of the bile is excreted each day, but the bulk of it is readsorbed and circulated back to the liver for reuse. When chitosan binds (attaches) to the bile acids, it carries them out with the feces, thus reducing the amount available for readsorption and recirculation. In order to produce more bile acids to make up this deficit, the body uses endogenous serum cholesterol since cholesterol is an essential component of bile. Supporting this hypothesis is the fact that a small clinical trial in which human patients were treated for hypercholesterolemia with chitosan showed that there was a definite increase in the amount of bile acids excreted with the ingestion of chitosan (Maezaki, Y. et al.).

Are There Any Adverse Side Effects?

- More of a caution than a side effect is the possibility that chitosan may also bind to fat-soluble vitamins and reduce the level of these in the body. This possibility has not yet been completely proven. However, it need not present a problem if daily supplementation with fat-soluble vitamins, at least two hours prior to consuming chitosan, is undertaken.

- To minimize the potential for constipation, it is necessary to drink at least 250 ml of water (a full glass is plenty) with every 1000 mg of product consumed. The amount of chitosan recommended to take per meal is usually 1000 mg. This should be taken with the meal, or meals, involving the most fat.

- Unless a person has an allergy to gelatin (chitosan is usually presented in gelatin capsules), it is unlikely that any allergic reaction will occur. Most allergic reactions to marine products involve proteins in the product, and there are no proteins in chitosan.

5

CANCER

This is such a complex disease with so many different types, causes, symptoms, and effects that it is quite inappropriate to attempt to discuss it in any detail in a book such as this. Under the general heading of cancer are tumors (malignant and benign), melanomas, lymphomas, and leukemias. The common factor in all of these forms of cancer is the *uncontrolled replication of cells*.

Cells are the body's basic units of life just as the letters of the alphabet are the basic units of a book. There are millions of cells of different types making up our body and carrying out the functions necessary for growth and life. These cells are constantly developing and dividing as the body requires them. Under normal circumstances, cells multiply and die off in an orderly fashion and at a controlled rate. Here is yet another example of balance being the key to health because cancer occurs when this orderly pattern veers out of balance. In cancer there is an abnormal growth of cells; that is, cells continue to grow and divide even though the body does not need them. Alternatively, the old cells do not die off when they have been replaced by new ones.

When there is uncontrolled cell growth in the body tissues, a mass of extra tissue forming a tumor develops. Lymphomas, of which there are many types, are tumors that occur as a result of abnormal cells in the lymphatic system. The lymphatic system is part of our immune defense mechanism, comprising tubes containing lymph fluid (a source of lymphocytes—white cells). Because lymph is carried to almost all parts of the body, the abnormal cells can spread to most organs and cause tumors (lymphomas) to develop. If the abnormal growth of cells occurs in the blood, it is the leukemia form of cancer that develops. In most cases of leukemia, it is also the abnormal development of white blood cells that creates the problem. These are our soldier cells, and because the abnormal cells are not able to function properly, the immune system is compromised, leading to inadequate resistance to disease.

All the causative factors for cancers are not completely understood. There is still divided opinion as to the relevance of genetic influences. However, the cause of some forms of cancer is believed to be a result of exposure to certain chemicals. Unfortunately, the list of chemicals being found to be carcinogenic is still growing. Other forms of cancer appear to be the result of a viral infection or overexposure to the ultraviolet rays in sunlight. An imbalance in the female hormones estrogen and progesterone have been implicated in breast and uterine cancers.

Treating Cancer: Help from the Sea

The potentially terminal nature of cancer makes it a highly emotive subject, and any treatment must be approached in a sensitive and responsible manner. To advocate unproven or ineffective treatments for commercial gain would have to be the worst example of charlatanism. The two most widely used, and in many cases the most effective, treatments for cancers in general are radiation therapy and chemotherapy. Both have unpleasant side effects such as hair loss, skin rashes, and weakened immunity. However, these effects can be temporary with full recovery occurring post-treatment and are often less of a problem than the disease itself.

Some of the most effective treatments to come from the sea are most likely to be derived from the marine sponges. These sedentary and unexciting-looking animals are proving to be a most prolific source of potential new anticancer treatments. Currently, it is estimated that at least 300 new potential anticancer substances derived from the marine sponges are being screened for possible use in drug therapy for cancer.

The introductory chapter of this book explained that the molecular structure of some of the bioactive, therapeutic compounds found in marine animals is too complex for us to commercially synthesize. The simple sea anemone was presented as an example. A similar situation applies to the sponges. Such is the case for one very promising new anticancer drug derived from a sponge found off the coast of New Zealand. In order to obtain sufficient product for the screening tests being conducted at the National Cancer Institute in the United States, it has been necessary to establish a marine farm in New Zealand to cultivate this species of sponge. Fortunately, given the appropriate temperature and salinity (salt content) of the seawater, sponges are relatively simple to cultivate.

The mechanism by which the products derived from sponges will treat cancer is likely to be a specific toxic action on the cancer cells (*cytotoxicity*) as contrasted with a relatively nontoxic action on normal cells. Also derived from the sea are two alternative products that have been used successfully to treat certain cancers and that have a different mechanism for attacking the disease. These alternative products are both derived from sharks, although there is a very important distinction between the type of shark that provides each product. In this chapter we will examine the information available on these two products and reference the sources of that information.

Deep Sea Shark Liver Oil

One of the products is deep sea shark liver oil, and the bioactive components are called *alkylglycerols* (also known as diacylglyceryl ethers and alkoxyglycerols). The important distinction between the sharks from which this oil is derived and those from which shark cartilage, the other product, is derived is the deep sea factor. Only species of deep sea shark have a liver oil specifically rich in alkyglycerols, whereas all sharks can provide the cartilage product.

It is important to point out here that the liver oil and the cartilage are by-products of the normal fishing industry; sharks are not caught specifically for their livers or their cartilage. In fact, these products used to be thrown away but are now able to be utilized for valuable therapeutic purposes. A further point to be noted is that shark meat is widely used for fish dishes. It is healthy, wholesome white fish meat, and sharks are fished, just as are other species, for their meat.

Alkylglycerols are found in relatively high concentration in our bone marrow, human breast milk, and deep sea shark liver oil. The main function of these compounds is enhancement of the immune system which, in our bodies, is initially derived from the bone marrow. In the breast-feeding mother, the innate immunity of the baby is introduced via the breast milk. More detail on the functioning of the human immune system and on deep sea shark liver oil follows in Chapter 6.

Numerous studies have been conducted on the application of alkylglycerols in cancer treatment and immunostimulation. It is only possible to refer to a few of these here. Most of the studies involving alkylglycerols, derived from deep sea shark liver oil, in the treatment of cancer were conducted on patients receiving radiation therapy for uterine cancer. Interestingly, it was found that the product proved to be most effective when used prophylactically as opposed to as post-radiation treatment (Brohult et al.). This is not surprising since prophylactic use of the alkylglycerols will build up and maintain healthy white cells.

It may be helpful here to quote directly from one of the published papers:

It is observed that
1. The incidence of injuries is considerably lower in the alkoxyglycerol groups than in the control group—especially for group 1 where alkoxy-glycerols have been administered prophylactically. The incidence of total injuries is reduced to about 50%.

2. Complex injuries are reduced to about 1/3 in the prophylactic group compared with the control group, i.e., the prophylactic administration of alkoxyglycerols has reduced the growth of the tumor.

3. Multiple injuries are less frequent in the prophylactic group compared with the control group (1.1% compared with 6.5%).

4. When alkoxyglycerols are administered only during and after radiation treatment, no effect is observed on the incidence of complex injuries, while a significant decrease is found for the injuries due to radiation only (22.8% to 8.9%).

5. The preliminary results from the double blind study, where the patients have been followed up for 3.5 years after the commencement of treatment, indicate that the prophylactic administration of alkoxyglycerols reduced the total incidence of injuries to about 50%.

In the discussion section of this paper the significance of using alkoxyglycerols as a prophylactic as opposed to their use as a remedial treatment is clearly defined.

The analysis of injuries of the bladder (and ureters) and rectum (and intestine) following intracavity and external radiation therapy for carcinoma of the uterine cervix has shown a marked decrease in the incidence of injuries in cases where alkoxyglycerols are administered. There are noticeable differences in effect, however, related to the schedule of administration of alkoxyglycerols, and related to whether the injury represents a pure radiation damage of the tissue or represents a combination of radiation injury and residual or recurrent tumor growth. The prophylactic treatment with alkoxyglycerols in combination with radiotherapy apparently prevents the development of radiation damage and the growth of the tumor, separately or combined. Nonprophylactic administration of alkoxyglycerols does not seem to influence the tumor growth—but still protects against radiation damage.

The mechanism for the antitumor (anticancer) activity of the alkoxyglycerols in deep sea shark liver oil is thought to be associated with the activation of cells called *macrophages* (Pugliease, P. et al., 1998). Macrophages are large cells in our immune system that are equipped to recognize and destroy invasive cells by engulfing them and carrying them out of our system. This is a very much simplified description of macrophages because they are a part of a highly regulated and very versatile immune cellular system. However, studies have clearly shown that the stimulation of macrophage activity by alkoxyglycerols is linked to a cytotoxic effect on tumor cells (Andreesen et al., 1978; Berdel et al., 1980; Modelell et al., 1979).

Shark Cartilage

The other cancer-related product to be derived from sharks is shark cartilage powder. The powder is a freeze-dried and fine-milled preparation of the backbones (these are actually cartilaginous structures rather than a true backbone) and gills of the shark that used to be thrown away as waste materials. It is good to see that a by-product of the fishing industry is now being utilized for a valuable purpose.

A significant amount of research has been conducted on the effect of shark cartilage as a possible treatment for cancer. Much of this research has been carried out in the United States, with some valuable laboratory evidence for the probable mechanism of action coming from research done in New Zealand.

Angiogenesis literally translates as "the birth of new blood vessels," and this process has been linked directly to the growth and spread (metastasis) of tumors (Weidner, M. D. et al., 1991). Tumors require new capillary blood vessels in order to grow and spread; therefore, the inhibition of angiogenesis should reduce or prevent the growth and spread of tumors. This has proven to be the case in a number of studies at the laboratory level (Lee, A. et al., 1983; D'Amore, P. A., 1988; Davis, P. F. et al., 1997). The fact that most of the work on angiogenesis inhibition as a potential control for tumor development and metastasis has been conducted at the laboratory level does not minimize its importance for human application since human tumors will involve the same parameters. In fact, clinical studies involving human subjects have already begun in the United States as a result of publicity on the effect of shark cartilage in cancer by Dr. William Lane (Lane, I. W. et al., 1992 & 1996).

Although not regarded as objective or clinical evidence, numerous anecdotal reports of success in stabilizing cancer and, in some cases reversing the progress, have been quoted. The author has personally received a significant number of unsolicited reports from people suffering a variety of forms of cancer for whom the regular screening has shown tumor stabilization or regression. This being the case, it would be reasonable to ask why there has not been a greater degree of success with these two products and why they are not a first-line treatment since they do not produce significant adverse side effects. The answer is that people have typically only tried these treatments as a last resort, after having gone through orthodox therapies without success. They are therefore very difficult cases with well-developed cancers that have resisted radiation and/or powerful chemotherapy. In fairness, it must be pointed out that a clinician faced with treating a patient for cancer needs to adopt the most proven and clinically established procedures available rather than a potentially effective, but new treatment, that has not yet been fully documented.

It would be quite wrong to suggest that deep sea shark liver oil or shark cartilage definitely provide the answer to this disease. Because it is such a highly emotive subject, people will grasp at anything purported to offer a chance of recovery. However, it would also be wrong to avoid discussing these alternatives to radiation and chemotherapy that might help, and are certainly worth a try if the other treatments have been unsuccessful.

6

THE COMMON COLD, INFLUENZA, AND VIRAL DISORDERS

This subject embraces those complaints we humans experience frequently. In the author's opinion, one of the surest ways to contract a viral disorder that can spread by the aerosol effect (sneezing and coughing) is to travel a long distance by aircraft. Here the viruses, sneezed or coughed into the air, are generously spread throughout the aircraft by the air-conditioning system. Many offices will also present a similar opportunity as a result of air-conditioning systems—an example of one of the less desirable features of our modern lifestyle. Of course, not all viral infections are spread in this way. Some, such as hepatitis B, require physical contact either by blood or saliva, whereas others, such as hepatitis A, are usually transmitted by contaminated foods, resulting from poor hygiene practices, in the same way that many bacterial diseases are contracted.

Because it is not possible to avoid the initial attack by the common cold or influenza virus, our only defense is to have a strong immune system that can deal with the virus once it is in our system. In this way we can minimize the symptoms that would normally follow the viral attack and significantly shorten the period of discomfort. We have been referring to an "attack" by the virus, and this is exactly what it is, our body has been subjected to an invasion by hostile forces. Our natural defenses will recognize this invasion and, under the right circumstances, will repel the attackers. Just as in human warfare, the outcome of this battle will depend on the relative strength of each of the forces, and this is related to the number of soldier cells we have available for action in our immune system. It might be helpful to the reader if, at this point, the basic features and functions of our immune system are briefly described.

The Human Immune System

The human immune system is designed to protect us from the harmful effects of our environment and disease-producing organisms, including bacteria, viruses, and other microbes. Without a well-developed and maintained immune system, we will suffer infections and serious, life-threatening diseases—all of which emphasizes improving our ability to fight off disease in order to maintain our overall health.

In humans, our immune system components are made up of the *lymph*, the *thymus*, and, of course, the *red bone marrow*. The white blood cells, which form the basis of the system, are called *leucocytes* or *white corpuscles*. The leucocytes themselves are divided into three classes, each of which has a special function in the immune system. They are: B lymphocytes, so called because they are located in the bone marrow; T lymphocytes, which, although they originate in the bone marrow, are located in the thymus gland; and the neutrophils (also known as polymorphonuclear leucocytes).

In general, the B lymphocytes are the antibody-producing cells; the T lymphocytes attend to cell-mediated immunity; and the neutrophils are involved in inflammatory-based activities.

In very loose terms, we can liken these classes of white cells to a nation's defense forces—the navy, army, and air force. In some instances only one of the three will be required to deal with an invasive situation, although there may be occasions where all three are required.

There are several types of immunity, and we soon develop these progressively after leaving the safety of our mother's womb. In fact, by the time we have reached maturity, we may well have four types protecting us to a greater or lesser extent.

We are born with a *natural immunity* derived in part from our parents, which renders us safe from certain diseases that would normally be fatal to other animal species. This form of immunity is our primary defense against anything the body considers to be alien. Unfortunately, there can be instances when our defense system will fail to recognize some nonalien substance and set about destroying it. This autoimmune response, where the body is literally attacking itself, is at the heart of a range of health problems now generally referred to as *autoimmune diseases*, including lupus and some forms of arthritis such as rheumatoid arthritis.

As we grow, we develop an *acquired immunity* through contracting diseases such as scarlet fever, measles, and others. Having contracted the disease, our body fights it by developing antibodies that attack and destroy the antagonist (*antigens*). Our immune system then has the antibodies on standby (or in reserve) in case it is exposed to another attack, in which case the disease does not have the opportunity to take hold.

Some immunities of this type are very long lasting, and once we have recovered from an attack of the disease we are then protected from any further attack for many years or even our lifetime.

An example of this is rubella. More commonly known as German measles, it is especially dangerous if contracted during pregnancy. However, if young girls contract the disease early in life, they are then protected by the immunity built up through exposure to the disease.

Today, because of the serious consequences to the unborn from Rubella, vaccination of young girls is encouraged to protect them from the disease. This form of immunity called *artificial immunity* is available for a range of serious illnesses, including Tuberculosis, Poliomyelitis, Diphtheria, and Whooping Cough.

Generally, there are two ways of acquiring artificial immunity. Through vaccination (also termed immunization), where the poison, virus, or bacteria (in a much weakened state) is introduced into the body by injection. Our immune system detects the invasion by a foreign substance and develops the antibodies to attack and destroy it. Generally, the process of vaccination involves gradually increasing the strength of the injected poison or bacteria so that we slowly build up an immunity strong enough to withstand a full-scale attack, should this be necessary. This type of artificial immunity is known as *active immunity* to differentiate it from *passive immunity*, both of which many of us will experience or have already experienced.

Passive immunity is obtained when the actual antibodies that fight the infection are injected directly into the body of someone who may be in danger of developing the disease. Normally the antibodies in the form of immunoglobulins will have been derived from another person or animal that has developed sufficient antibodies or antitoxins specific to the disease, such as Tetanus (also known as Lockjaw).

To obtain the antibodies needed, a weakened form of the disease is injected into a person or animal so that they will develop antibodies or antitoxins to the disease. This part of the operation is the same as that for active immunity. The difference is that when the at-risk person who has not been previously immunized is injected with antibody-containing serum from the immunized animal or person, they receive the antibodies needed to defend them against the disease.

This method has proved highly successful in treating or preventing a range of illnesses. The serums produced by this technique are called *antiserums* and are in common use for the treatment of tetanus poisoning, snake venom poisoning, botulism, and some other infections.

The Sea in the Prevention of Viral Infections

It may seem strange that, in spite of the major differences between humans and the shark, something derived from this marine animal can have such a positive and beneficial effect on the human immune system. It should not be too surprising since, historically, we have used fish oils such as cod liver oil and halibut liver oil for protection from winter colds for many years. Properly processed, these fish liver oils are effective stimulants for our immune system, but not as effective as deep sea shark liver oil. The reason for the difference is in the amount of the components that are specifically responsible for stimulation of the immune system in the different oils.

In the shark, the components of the immune system are found in the liver. Sharks do not have bone marrow. In fact they do not have bones at all, but a cartilage equivalent to our backbone. If the livers from certain species of shark are carefully preserved at the time of capture, the oil from these livers will contain valuable compounds that have a profound influence on the health and strength of our human immune system. Only certain species of shark (actually they are large dogfish, but they belong to the shark family in the same way that skates and rays do) produce the liver oil with these properties, and these are the species that live in very deep, cold waters. The main regions where these sharks are caught are the Atlantic Ocean and the South Pacific Ocean.

How can deep sea shark liver oil influence the health and strength of our complex immune system? Basically, by increasing or maintaining the number of our white blood cells. This is, in effect, similar to increasing the number of combatants employed in the armed forces mentioned previously.

We are enhancing our immunity against invasion by building a stronger army of soldiers or leucocytes. Provided that our immune system is able to recognize the alien cells that are invading, it will immediately mobilize the necessary immune forces to attack and immobilize the invaders.

Therefore, just as is the case with our navy, army, or air force, the number of troops and their degree of readiness is important to our security. In the case of the immune system, we are more at risk of infection if our white blood cell count is lower than normal. Of course, even with a very strong immune system, we cannot prevent an invasion by bacteria or viruses. What we do achieve is a rapid mobilization of our defenses to counter the invasion and a very much shortened period of suffering the discomfort and symptoms of the particular infection.

The components in deep sea shark liver oil that provide this immune-boosting function are the *alkylglycerols*. The naturally occurring alkylglycerols found in deep sea shark liver oil are a group of compounds in which the basic glycerol molecule has had a hydrogen atom substituted by alcohols as illustrated below.

Glycerol	Alkylglycerol
CH_2-OH	CH_2-OH-R^*
$\mid$	$\mid$
CH_2-OH	$CH-OH$
$\mid$	$\mid$
CH_2-OH	CH_2-OH

*In deep sea shark liver oil, R = Chimyl, Batyl, or Selachyl Alcohol.

At least one mechanism by which the alkylglycerols influence our immune system was established during research on immune stimulation in mice (Yamamoto et al., 1998). This work indicated that small amounts of alkylglycerols stimulated macrophage activity. Macrophages are white cells that could be classed as our first line of defense against invading viruses. The macrophage first detects the attacking virus and consumes it. Then it displays pieces of the virus (these are called antigens) on its surface so that the lymphocytes (our soldier cells) can identify the enemy antigen. Our T lymphocytes then attack the viruses and stimulate our B lymphocytes to produce antibodies that attach to the antigens on the viruses and make it easier for the macrophages to consume and destroy them. All of this warfare produces a substance called *complement* that envelops the destroyed viruses and carries them out of our system as a form of mucus that we call phlegm. We can therefore appreciate that stimulation of our macrophages is an important form of defense against viral infection, similar, in fact, to keeping a nation's defense forces fit and ready in case of an invasion.

In another research project, in which alkylglycerols influenced the destruction of cancer cell membranes by a reaction known as *oxidative burst*, it was established that the alkylglycerols induced this reaction via an iron-induced lipid peroxidation reaction (Wagner et al., 1992). Interestingly, only the cancer cells in the test were affected; normal cells were not affected. For a number of reasons this was an important finding since oxidative reactions in general are undesirable. However, the significance of this work for our immune defense discussion is that oxidative bursts play an important role in providing our bactericidal and antiviral protection via the activity of other white cells, the neutrophils.

A much earlier study also had shown a positive influence of the alkylglycerols in deep sea shark liver oil on immune stimulation. This study was particularly concerned with one specific group of the alkylglycerols called *methoxy-substituted alkylglycerols.* We need not be concerned with the chemistry of the difference here since the methoxy-substituted alkylglycerols (also called methoxy-substituted glycerol ethers) naturally comprise about 3 percent of the alkylglycerols in deep sea shark liver oil (Boeryd et al., 1978). In this study it was shown that oral administration of the oil stimulated T-lymphocyte function, and it was postulated that the influence may occur right at the heart of the immune system—in the bone marrow.

An important point to note about deep sea shark liver oil is that it should be used prophylactically, not as a treatment once the infection has been encountered. The author, although philosophically not a pill-taking person, will not miss taking a 1000-mg capsule of this product each day. The benefit of this supplementation has been demonstrated many times over the past five years when young, healthy work colleagues have succumbed to bouts of influenza or the common cold, leading to days off work and much discomfort. At the same time, the author, who has been exposed to all the same bacteria or viruses, has not missed a workday—but has missed the misery of the cold and influenza symptoms!

Note: It is important when consuming fish oils to be aware that these oils normally contain the oil-soluble vitamins A and D. While we need these vitamins for good health, it is important that we are not exposed to excessive amounts, as these can be toxic. Some fish oils contain toxic levels of vitamin A in particular and have to be diluted for human consumption. Some of the surface-dwelling sharks have liver oils that contain high levels of vitamin A. However, deep sea shark liver oil does not contain large amounts of either vitamin A or D and is quite safe to consume. In this respect, it is important to note that other components of the diet, such as carrots and green leaf vegetables, are also a source of vitamin A, and sunshine or fortified milk can provide vitamin D.

The recommended daily allowance for vitamin A is 1000 retinol equivalents per day and for vitamin D is 400 International Units (IU). The deep sea shark liver oil referred to in this book has a vitamin A level less than 400 retinol equivalents per daily dose of 1000 mg, with vitamin D being barely detectable in this amount.

7

DERMATOLOGICAL

DISEASES

Dermatological diseases are those that involve inflammation of the skin. There are many such diseases with different causes and different names. Only a general description of each of the three principal types—dermatitis, eczema, and psoriasis—can be addressed in a little book such as this because comprehensive coverage of these diseases would occupy complete books in their own right. Also, it is not easy to distinguish between dermatitis and eczema because both are a result of skin sensitivity to an external irritant and they may only be different terms for the same complaint.

Dermatitis

Basically, this term covers situations where contact between the skin and an external substance, to which the skin is sensitive or allergic, causes redness, skin eruptions, and inflammation. A wide range of substances can create this situation, including clothing fabrics, cosmetics, plants, and antibiotics. Even the sun can create dermatitis in individuals who are photosensitive, taking the form of a more extensively damaged skin condition than that of ordinary sunburn. Some drugs can cause a person to become photosensitive and thus susceptible to this type of dermatitis. Just as with other allergies, what causes a dermatological reaction in one person may have absolutely no effect on others.

The usual treatment for dermatitis is the use of a cooling, skin-covering substance such as calamine lotion, if the condition is not too severe. In more severe cases corticosteroids that attack the inflammatory components of the condition are used.

Eczema

This disease is characterized by the reaction of the skin to irritants resulting in skin eruptions that break down to ooze fluids. Severe itching is a problem, sometimes causing the sufferer to scratch until an extensive area of the body is bleeding. If there is a differentiating factor between dermatitis and eczema, it is that, in eczema, there is probably a constitutional element involved that renders the person susceptible to a skin allergy response. The eruption and oozing of pus that accompanies a burn is a form of eczema that can spread rapidly and that needs special care and treatment.

The usual treatment for eczema is, not surprisingly, similar to that for dermatitis. Depending on the specific situation, it consists of topical application of steroids, calamine lotion, and, in the case of burns or wounds, sometimes antibiotics.

Psoriasis

Although the symptoms of psoriasis are similar to those of the other dermatological diseases, the causative factors are different. Psoriasis is a skin disorder for which the basic cause is uncontrolled cell growth leading to a proliferation of new blood vessels and an accelerated skin-cell life cycle. It is an inflammatory disorder that frequently occurs during adolescence but can also occur in adult life. While it is not a contagious disease, it can be unsightly and a deterrent to close physical contact. This, coupled with the fact that it can also be brought on by depression, can lead to a vicious cycle and considerable distress for the person affected. The symptoms of psoriasis manifest in itchy, rough, scaly areas of the skin, and it is these that bleed when the scale is removed by scratching. The face and scalp are particularly susceptible to psoriatic eruptions although these may first occur on the arms and legs.

Since psoriasis is an inflammatory condition, treatment is usually with anti-inflammatory preparations such as ointments containing corticosteroids. Usually, it is also necessary to treat the condition that is responsible for the psoriasis, particularly if this is a rheumatic or depressive condition.

The Sea in the Treatment of Dermatological Diseases

From the above, it can be seen that to effectively treat these diseases we need a combination of anti-inflammatory, anti-angiogenic, and immunomodulatory agents. The anti-inflammatory activity will help by inhibiting the production of pro-inflammatory compounds called leukotrienes. A particular group of leukotrienes are known to be adversely influential in inflammatory and allergic reactions such as asthma. By inhibiting the endogenous (within our own body) biosynthesis of these compounds, the dilation of skin capillaries—one of the causes of psoriatic eruptions—is prevented.

Angiogenesis was referred to in Chapter 5, but there is no harm in redefining this function here. As the name implies, *angiogenesis* means "the birth or development of new blood vessels." Under normal circumstances this is a controlled function and does not create problems. However, under some circumstances angiogenesis gets out of control and results in a proliferation of new blood vessels that are not needed. This is the case in psoriasis where the combined effect of inflammation and angiogenesis creates the redness, eruptions, and irritation at the skin surface.

Immunomodulation simply means influencing the immune system. It can mean strengthening the immune system to combat disease organisms such as viruses, but it can also mean damping down the immune system to reduce the response where this is desirable—for example, to an inflammatory stimulus. Because dermatological disorders can involve autoimmune reactions, an immunomodulatory agent can help reduce this effect.

A New Zealand product that contains deep sea shark liver oil and shark cartilage as the active components in a topical cream has been shown to be beneficial in rapidly relieving the itching and more slowly reducing the redness and scaly skin eruptions associated with these disorders. The vitamins A and D, although present in the cream, are at very low levels and vitamin E is present only as an added antioxidant for the oils.

In local trials of the product, one patient had previously suffered so severely that she would scratch in her sleep until her bedsheets would be covered in blood in the morning. In describing her experience with the cream, she said that it took four days before she awoke in the morning to find no blood on the bedsheets and no irritating itch. Provided that she applied the cream twice each day, this condition was maintained. She did note, however, that during a particularly stressful period at work, she needed an additional application of the cream during the day. Another woman reported that the itching on her arms and legs eased within an hour of applying the cream, and the redness and scaliness disappeared after about a week. However, if she did not apply the cream each day, the symptoms returned. An interesting report came from a male patient who was the supervisor at a seafood processing plant. He had become extremely sensitized to certain seafood products and would develop a severe and itchy rash on his scalp and arms if in the vicinity of areas where these were being processed. Within a week of applying the cream on a daily basis, his scalp and arms were completely clear!

The mechanism by which this marine product achieves these results is almost certainly a combination of the immunomodulatory function of the deep sea shark liver oil with the anti-inflammatory and angiogenesis inhibitory functions of the shark cartilage. There is also an added benefit derived from the natural content of squalene in the deep sea shark liver oil. This is due to the emollient and mild bactericidal functions of this compound that will aid in the recovery of skin health and protect against bacterial infection during the healing process. The fact that this cream can be applied directly to the affected areas, be rapidly absorbed, and produce early symptomatic relief is yet another example of the value of marine, natural therapeutic treatments for widespread and distressing disorders.

8

HYPERLIPIDEMIA

Hyperlipidemia is the name that is generally used for a condition in which a person's cholesterol level is too high. More accurately, it describes a condition where the total level of fats is too high. This can be a serious condition and, unfortunately, is a relatively common one, particularly where a diet high in saturated fats is combined with a sedentary lifestyle. Hyperlipidemia is commonly associated with cardiovascular diseases such as heart failure and other serious problems of the cardiovascular system that can result in sudden death. It is therefore a condition that warrants careful attention.

We need fats in our diet because they provide us with a reserve energy source and also many of the essential components for our bodily functions. However, a diet that is too high in the saturated fats and not high enough in the unsaturated ones can lead to a range of disease states, including diabetes mellitus, high blood pressure, and coronary thrombosis.

There is a tendency to consider fats as either "good" or "bad," but this is not really an accurate classification because most of them can be *either* good or bad depending on the amount ingested and the function they perform. What is really needed for good health is a balance of dietary fats combined with a balance of physical exercise. Note the word *balance* again—this is really the key to success in everything, including our health. It is also one of the reasons why the saltwater bodies are so valuable as mentioned in the first chapter. The seas comprise the most ecologically and nutritionally balanced medium we have on our planet Earth!

Vegetable and animal fats and oils come under the general term *lipids*: Those lipids having a high degree of unsaturation are oils and those with a high degree of saturation are fats and waxes. One of the lipids with a high degree of saturation is cholesterol, and it is now well known that a high cholesterol level in our blood is undesirable because it can lead to the diseases mentioned earlier. Strictly speaking, cholesterol is a lipoprotein (i.e., a combination of lipid and protein), and it is an essential component of our body with several very important roles to play.

Cholesterol is widely distributed throughout our body because it forms a vital part of the cell membranes. In addition, cholesterol is a natural component of our blood and is essential for the production of our sex hormones and our bile acids. Other functions performed by dietary fats in general include: facilitating the digestion of important nutrients, suppressing our appetite, and providing the raw material for our sebaceous glands to produce the lubricant that maintains our skin health.

There are two sources for the cholesterol in our body. One is dietary—meats, dairy products, and some types of fish contain cholesterol. Meats contain the highest amounts of cholesterol while only a few species of fish (mainly shrimp, squid, and abalone) contain reasonably high levels. Most fish and shellfish are low in cholesterol content. The highest levels are contained in the edible animal organs such as liver. The other (internal) source is our own liver, which manufactures cholesterol for the essential functions mentioned earlier. Vegetables do not contain any cholesterol.

Under the right conditions of diet and exercise, the levels of cholesterol in our blood from the combined sources will match that required for healthy metabolism and will not create health problems. Of course this level varies from individual to individual, and in some instances a higher than normal cholesterol level can be due to genetic factors rather than diet.

There are two forms of cholesterol in our body and, for health purposes, it is the ratio of the two forms that is possibly more important than the total amount. The two forms are known as *low-density lipoprotein* (LDL) and *high-density lipoprotein* (HDL). These names derive from the fact that cholesterol has to combine with some special proteins called lipoproteins (because they are a combination of a lipid and a protein) in order to dissolve in the blood. The low- or high-density factor relates to the number of protein molecules attached to the lipid. The higher the number of protein molecules, the higher the density of the cholesterol molecule. Of the two forms, it is LDL cholesterol that presents the greater health risk since it is this form that causes the deposit of cholesterol plaque on the arterial walls. Whether this feature of LDL is due to the smaller size of the LDL molecules (as compared with HDL cholesterol), allowing them to penetrate the endothelial cell wall of the artery, or whether, as seems more likely, it is because they are more susceptible to oxidation than their HDL counterparts, is not certain.

Nevertheless, the fact is that it is desirable to have a high HDL to LDL cholesterol ratio rather than the other way round. HDL cholesterol is often referred to as the *good* cholesterol because it performs the function of reducing the amount of LDL cholesterol accumulated on the arterial walls by interfering with the deposition process and also by removing deposited cholesterol and carrying this to the liver for processing into bile.

The Sea in the Treatment of Hyperlipidemia

There has been a great deal of publicity given to the beneficial effect of the *omega-3 fatty acids* in reducing the incidence of heart disease. As with many important discoveries, serendipity played a major role in that it was noted that the Eskimo race, which has a diet that is very high in fats, did not suffer the same level of cardiac problems and associated deaths as did other races. The answer to this apparent aberration came with the discovery that, although Eskimos were consuming a diet high in fats, the diet was also very high in its omega-3 fatty-acid content. This diet, because it was rich in omega-3 fatty acids, played a prophylactic role in preventing the buildup of cholesterols and fatty plaques rather than a treatment role. Prevention of a disease state is always preferable to the treatment of one.

The mechanism by which omega-3 fatty acids reduce the risk of heart disease is probably that of interfering with the production of a group of prostaglandins called thromboxanes. We have already met the prostaglandins in earlier chapters so I will not describe them again here. However, this particular group of thromboxanes is responsible for promoting the clumping of platelets in the blood. This is a necessary function for blood clotting in the event of injury. However, as with all other bodily functions, it is again a matter of balance. Thromboxanes are important in blood-platelet clumping, but another group of prostaglandins called prostacyclins are present to moderate this activity. In the presence of omega-3 fatty acids, the production of the clumping thromboxane is reduced, and this reduces the potential for clumps of cells to form blood clots, particularly in the presence of serum cholesterol. By maintaining a healthy arterial system, the risk of blood clots and elevated blood-pressure levels is avoided.

Oils and fats also contain a group of compounds called *triglycerides*. Speaking very generally, these provide, in addition to certain essential pharmacological functions, our energy store and thermal insulation. They are therefore essential ingredients of our diet. However, it is important to utilize the triglycerides (burn them off) in exercise so that their level does not become too high where they can cause a type of heart disease called ischemic heart disease. In very simple terms, this is a condition where the body is starved of blood due to blockage of arteries (thrombosis).

Seafoods provide the best source of omega-3 fatty acids, as well as having the lowest levels of cholesterol among the three foodstuffs containing cholesterol (meats, including poultry; dairy

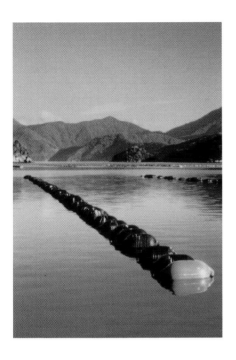

New Zealand Green-Lipped
Mussel Farm, courtesy of
Healtheries, NZ Ltd.

New Zealand Green-Lipped
Mussel Stack, courtesy of
Healtheries, NZ Ltd.

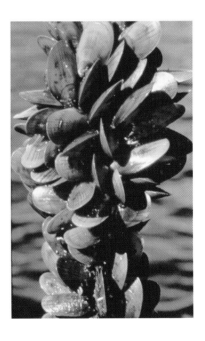

The photographs on the following two pages were taken
by *Ian Skipworth*. Brilliant pink sea anemones *(left page)*.
Living sea coral *(right page)*.

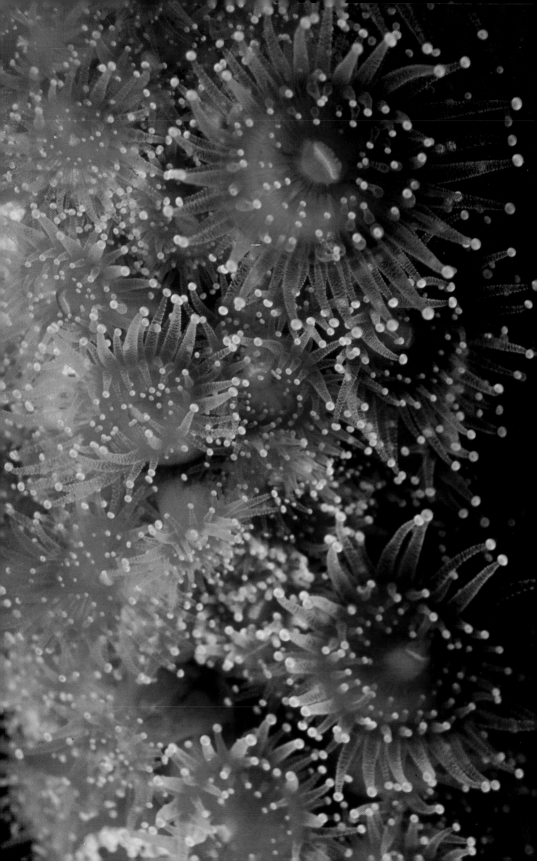

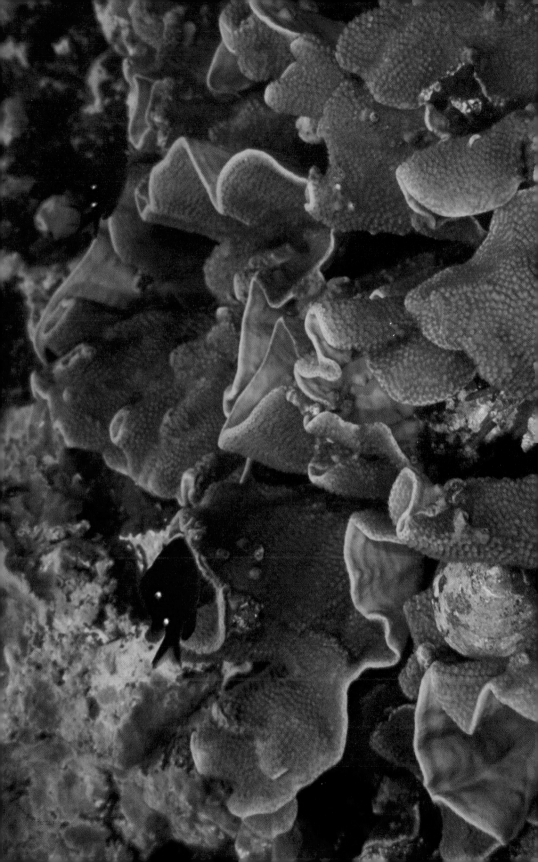

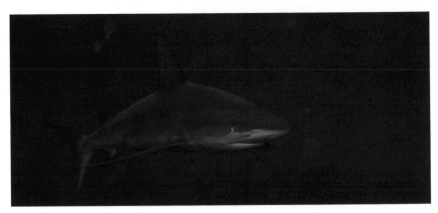

Reef shark, source of shark cartilage.
Photo by *Ian Skipworth.*

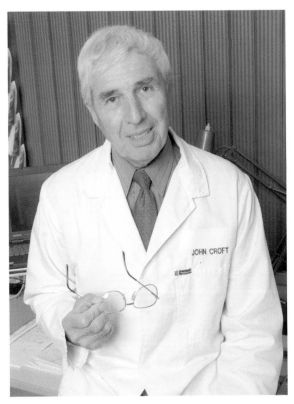

John Croft, LRSC, MRSNZ, FRSH.
Photo by *Richard Simpson.*

foods; and fish). Therefore, a diet containing a sufficient content of seafood will provide a significant preventative effect against heart disease. However, if a seafood diet is inconvenient or unpalatable, the same benefit can be obtained by consuming a high-quality omega-3 product in the form of fish-oil capsules. The two most common omega-3 fatty acids present in fish oils are eicosapentaenoic acid (EPA) and docosahexaenoic acid (DHA). These are usually present in these levels in high-quality fish oils: 18 percent EPA and 12 percent DHA. It is possible to find different ratios in certain fish oils (tuna is an example where this ratio is reversed), and even to modify the ratios, but for the purpose of arterial and heart health the 18/12 ratio is satisfactory. Other ratios will be discussed in a later chapter where they have application to a different condition.

Numerous studies have been conducted into the effects of the omega-3 fatty acids on heart disease, and there is now plenty of scientific and clinical evidence to support the fact that regular consumption of these fatty acids will reduce the possibility of contracting heart disease. In addition to studies on the cholesterol-lowering functions of the omega-3 fatty acids, other studies have demonstrated the ability of these compounds to reduce the level of triglycerides circulating in the bloodstream. Just another example of a natural product from one balanced medium, the sea, helping to restore the balance in another vital medium, our bloodstream.

The sea also provides a treatment for those whose serum cholesterol is too high in a product called beta-chitosan. This product, as we will see, has the ability to significantly lower serum cholesterol levels without causing the unpleasant side effects that are associated with the group of drugs used for this purpose. The difference from the omega-3 fatty acids is that we are now looking at a treatment as opposed to a preventative. Both have a role to play, however, in preventing the serious consequences of cardiac problems.

We have already met chitosan in the chapter dealing with atherosclerosis, but we are now looking at a different mechanism by which it functions to lower blood cholesterol levels.

The production of beta-chitosan from squid pens has been referred to in Chapter 4. It is this same beta-chitosan that functions as a cholesterol-lowering agent. As a result of the process that converts chitin to chitosan, called deacetylation because it involves the removal of acetyl groups from the chitin molecule as shown in the figure below, the chitosan molecule has a positive charge. For those who have not been exposed to science or the principles of electrostatic and magnetic forces, it will be helpful to know that two items with the same charge will repel each other, but two items with opposite charges will attract each other. Try this with two magnets, each of which will have a positive charge at one end and a negative charge at the other. The attractive force of the two ends with opposite charges will easily be detected.

The positive charge on the chitosan molecule will attract molecules with a negative charge in the same way. Fats tend to be negatively charged and therefore chitosan attracts these and binds to them. The resulting combined molecule of fat plus chitosan is too large to be absorbed by the cells lining the digestive tract and so it passes out of the body bound up in the stool. In this way less cholesterol (as well as other fats) gets into the bloodstream.

The negatively charged fats bind to these positively charged sites on the chitosan molecule.

Chitosan is a white powder that requires an acidic environment in which to dissolve. The stomach provides this acidic environment naturally and therefore it is only necessary to consume chitosan powder, normally in the form of gelatin capsules, just prior to a meal in order to get the benefit. When using chitosan, it is important to drink plenty of water. This has the effect of reducing the possibility of experiencing constipation and also helps to flush the system to clear wastes.

Numerous studies have been conducted on the cholesterol-lowering properties of chitosan; typically, these have shown that, among other things, chitosan is able to bind with several times its own weight of fats. One study, specifically measuring the binding action of chitosan with bile lipids, showed a 4 to 5 times binding capacity (Nauss et al., 1983), but it can be significantly greater than this when total fats are considered. In addition, and possibly of equal importance, other studies have shown that consumption of chitosan significantly enhanced the HDL to LDL ratio in human patients (Maezaki et al., 1993).

At the time of this writing, a study is just about to commence in New Zealand, and it will be the largest double-blind clinical trial undertaken to date. This trial will investigate the effects of beta-chitosan on the cholesterol levels, fat excretion, and reduction of obesity in 250 patients over a period of six months. The trial is to be conducted by the Clinical Trials Research Unit of the University of Auckland with the results being submitted for publication in one of the international, peer-reviewed medical journals.

Cautions for the Use of Chitosan

Although there have been no unpleasant side effects recorded with the use of chitosan, there are certain cautions that should be adopted. It has already been mentioned that plenty of water should accompany the taking of chitosan (at least one full 250-ml glass for each 1000 mg of beta-chitosan consumed). This will reduce the possibility of experiencing constipation.

Because it is not yet certain whether consumption of chitosan will deplete the level of the body's fat-soluble vitamins, it is advisable to supplement the diet with these vitamins when using chitosan. They should be taken at least two hours before chitosan is taken to allow time for absorption into the system.

This may seem like a rather obvious caution, but it is not advisable for a person with too low a cholesterol level (hypolipidemia) to use chitosan.

9

MENTAL

HEALTH

There are at least fifty different disorders and problems that fit under the all-embracing heading of mental health. It would not be possible, or appropriate, to attempt to offer informed comment on all of these in this book. Some mental disorders require surgical or intensive drug therapy to adequately treat the symptoms. However, the symptoms of others can be alleviated, or their development possibly prevented, by appropriate nutrition. In this chapter we will review some of the more common disorders, those that affect the most people, and see how natural products from the sea can help to alleviate the symptoms. Some of these mental disorders are associated with the aging process. However, some are most decidedly linked to stress-induced factors of modern-day living, peer pressure, and, unrelated as it may seem, the current level and speed of communication.

The reader may question how the speed of communication can possibly influence stress levels in the human being. There are several ways in which this influence occurs. For example, one pressure that now influences almost all those involved in international business is e-mail communication. Because this form of communication is so fast, it is possible to respond to customer questions immediately, and this is expected. However, sometimes it is helpful to have time to carefully consider the appropriate response to difficult questions. Prior to e-mail and telefax communication, this time could be taken without upsetting the customer who now, in the absence of a rapid e-mail response, may suspect that all is not well! While this may seem to be an unusual cause of stress, it is one cause that can be linked directly to the rapid speed of modern communication.

Other examples can be cited. For instance, on our television screens we now regularly watch natural disasters, even those that are happening in other countries, as they are actually taking place. We visit war zones in the midst of action and witness graphic details of the effects of real-life drought and famine. For most people, not only those who are particularly sensitive, this can be a stressful experience. Prior to the technology that allows this immediate transmission, often highly graphic, of distressing events right into our living rooms, we would not experience the horror of the stark visual images complementing the sound. In many instances we would be quite unaware of stress-causing incidents if they were remote. Hence, modern technology has resulted in a more stressful environment that, for some, has a detrimental effect on their mental health.

Another unfortunate factor that has resulted from our modern lifestyle is the increase in juvenile depression. Peer pressure can stem from such diverse areas as designer clothing and educational standards. The difficulty in finding rewarding employment on completion of education can have a significant depressing influence on many young people and, of course, the seriously depressing effects of drug abuse affect so many unfortunate young adults.

In some instances, the changes involved in puberty and adolescence alone are sufficient to cause, or at least exacerbate, depression in a young person.

The three types of mental illness that we consider in this chapter are *depression, decreased mental acuity,* and *age-related mental degeneration.* Of these, depression is probably the most widespread disorder, affecting up to 10 percent of the population at one time or another. Fortunately, however, depression is usually treatable and is one condition that products from the sea can greatly help.

There are several types of depression—fortunately now recognized as a genuine clinical disorder for which advice to "snap out of it" is not an appropriate treatment. Childhood depression and juvenile depression can affect those who are very young, right through to the developing adult. In the adult population, examples include: general depression (such as that caused by low self-esteem), manic depression (now known as a bipolar disorder), premenstrual and menopausal depression, and age-related depression. People who have suffered a stroke or a heart attack often tend to experience periods of depression following their recovery.

Symptoms of Depression

Whatever the cause of a depressive illness, many of the symptoms are the same, and it is worthwhile mentioning a few of the more common ones here. Some of these symptoms will be caused by changes in brain activities due to such things as diminished blood supply, inadequate nutrition influencing neurotransmission functions, and other factors. However, it is not uncommon for these initial symptoms to then lead to additional symptoms not directly related to the initial physiological activity. For example, difficulty in concentration and memory loss, coupled with the fatigue and lack of energy resulting from insomnia, can easily lead to a feeling of hopelessness, irritability, and pessimism. If, in turn, this leads to avoidance by friends or workmates, the situation might result in overeating with consequential physical problems. Some of the common symptoms of depression are:

- pessimism and feelings of worthlessness or hopelessness

- irritability and intolerance

- memory and decision-making difficulties

- insomnia with resulting tiredness and lack of energy

- potential for overeating, with subsequent obesity exacerbating depression

- physical problems such as persistent headaches and other pains.

The encouraging factor in all of this is that most of these symptoms can be successfully treated with either drug or alternative therapies.

Brain Functions and Depression

Without delving into the enormous complexity of our neurological mechanisms, it may be helpful to understand, in very general terms, some of the neurological functions that can lead to depression. One such function is a depleted serotonin level. Serotonin is an amino acid [5-hydroxytryptamine (5-HT)] that is very important for the regulation of neural transmissions. It is produced naturally in the body from endogenous *tryptophan* by the action of a specific enzyme. The enzymic process converts tryptophan to a compound called 5-hydroxytryptophan as an intermediary on the way to producing serotonin. The compound 5-hydroxytryptophan (abbreviated to 5-HTP) can also provide several other valuable functions that benefit the depressive disorders in mental health. Examples of a few of these functions are: alleviation of major and reactive depression, alleviation of panic disorder, alleviation of insomnia, reduction of anxiety, and reduction of appetite for people suffering obesity (Van Hiel et al., 1980; Den Boer et al., 1990; Sourlairac et al., 1977; Kahn et al., 1995; Cangiono et al., 1992).

In the human body most of the serotonin content is in the intestine where it influences intestinal motility. It also has an influence on the cardiovascular system. Our interest is in its function in mood and depression and this is linked to the effect of serotonin in stimulating nerve endings and neural transmissions. However, too high a level of serotonin in the body is not desirable since it may have an influence in the development of migraine headaches due to its effect on the vascular system. Fortunately, dietary serotonin is not well absorbed from the gastrointestinal tract and is rapidly metabolized in the body. If there is a deficiency of this important compound at any of the active sites where it is needed, the deficiency is made up by our internal biosynthesis system using dietary tryptophan. Under normal circumstances, provided that an adequate supply of tryptophan is available, this is a naturally regulated system.

Another important amino acid for healthy brain function is *tyrosine*. In common with other amino acids, two forms of tyrosine exist (L and D, which are simple mirror images of each other). It is the L form that our bodies utilize and this is the form that is found in foods. L-tyrosine is classed as a nonessential amino acid. This simply means that it can be synthesized naturally in the body from another amino acid and therefore is not normally needed to be provided from the diet. However, some people have a deficiency in tyrosine due to the inability of their body to synthesize it from the precursor amino acid phenylalanine. The function of L-tyrosine in relation to mental health is that it acts as a precursor for the production of the important neurotransmitters dopamine, epinephrine, and norepinephrine. When the brain level of these is enhanced by the availability of an increased level of L-tyrosine, more transmitter molecules are released by the neurons, resulting in increased neurotransmission activity. A benefit of L-tyrosine in providing a precursor for the biosynthesis of neurotransmitters is that it tends to be specific for the neurotransmitters that are responsible for stimulating the nerve impulses that help prevent depression.

A considerable amount of research has been carried out on the therapeutic effects of tyrosine in relation to mental health and its associated problems. The amino acid has been shown to be beneficial, among other things, for the relief of anxiety, the treatment of depression and mood, and the relief of stress

(Erdmann, R. et al., 1987; Gelenberg, A. J. et al., 1980; Brown, D. et al., 1999; Braverman, E. R., 1997; Bandaret, L. E., 1989; Deijen et al., 1994; Mai, C. A. et al., 1989; Reinstein, D. K. et al., 1985).

From reading the previous paragraphs, it would seem reasonable to assume that it would be beneficial for someone suffering depression to consume plenty of tryptophan and L-tyrosine. This is not generally the case, and would be undesirable since both can have significant adverse effects. However, a balanced level of each is essential for healthy brain and antidepressant function and, if the body cannot produce these itself due to the lack of the necessary enzymes, then appropriate dietary supplementation can provide the solution in many cases.

While tryptophan is not readily available from regularly consumed marine sources (dairy products will be the most natural source for this compound), tyrosine and its precursor phenylalanine are readily available, in particular in shellfish. The rich content of amino acids in marine sources such as shellfish makes a valuable contribution to the nutrient balance required for healthy mental function. For those unable to consume shellfish or appropriate dairy products regularly, a product that combines the functional derivatives of these can provide a useful alternative.

Aging, Mental Acuity, and Brain Health

At some time or another everyone suspects that mental acuity may be deteriorating, and I am sure that one of the feelings most common to all of us is that of memory failure. Neither of these experiences is necessarily due to deteriorating brain functions. They can easily be related to such everyday factors as tiredness or having too many things happening at once. However, it is a fact that mental acuity and memory competence can decline with inadequate brain nutrition and also with the aging process.

In many instances, this decline can be retarded and possibly reversed by appropriate dietary intervention. Our brain needs nourishment just like our other body organs, and while the body is capable of manufacturing some of the nutritional components needed for healthy and efficient functioning of the brain, the raw materials for this manufacture must be supplied in the form of the foods we eat. There are some nutrients that the body is unable to manufacture itself and these must be provided directly by the diet. These nutrients are distinguished by the designation *essential*. Examples are the essential amino acids and essential fatty acids.

The proteins we eat provide the amino acids needed for the production of our neurotransmitters, vital components of our neurons, which, among other things, perform the controlling functions for mental activities such as mood and anxiety. The fats we eat are vital for the production and maintenance of the cell membranes in the brain. About 60 percent of the brain is comprised of fat, and the composition of dietary fats that we provide for the body to biosynthesize or supply directly to the brain is very important. It is now recognized that the fats supplied to prenatal babies by their mothers during pregnancy can have a significant influence on the mental development and functioning of the child.

Aging and the Decline of Mental Acuity and Brain Health

It is not a foregone conclusion that the aging process must result in a decline in memory capability or sharpness of our mental abilities. Each of us probably knows an elderly person who has an active and sharp mind with surprising powers of recall. However, certain functions of our brain that are related to the aging process can result in memory difficulties and the inability to resolve mental challenges quickly. The mechanisms of these aging processes include our brain cell membranes losing their flexibility and an imbalance of brain cell metabolism and destruction caused by free-radical damage.

As a child and in our youth we have the ability and capacity to learn and absorb knowledge quickly. A striking example is how quickly and easily young refugee children learn a new language when taken to live in a country other than their own.

Often their parents will continue to have language difficulties many years after arrival in the new country, but the children will speak fluently and sound like their indigenous contemporaries. Why should this occur if there is no underlying disorder?

There are, of course, several possible reasons. However, one common reason is changes in the brain cell membrane structure. The membrane is the outer layer (equivalent to our skin) of a cell. In some cells its main function is to hold the contents of the cell together. In the neurons of the brain it has a far more dynamic function in that it regulates the transmission of messages, in the form of electrical impulses, between neurons. These messages are responsible for the functioning of our mind and body, so it is important that they are able to get through the system with minimal interference. One important requirement for the integrity of the neuron membrane is that it is strong but also very flexible. As we age we tend to lose some of the flexibility of our brain cell membranes and this interferes with the transmission of signals, not only to memory and acuity sites, but also to other organs in the body. Hence we also tend to slow down in our physical movements as we get older.

Although the brain needs a good supply of oxygen in order to function efficiently, paradoxically, a significant adverse effect on brain cell health is caused by oxidative damage. Oxidative damage is caused by free radicals, unstable chemical molecules that damage cell membranes by changing the nature of the fatty acid components. During much of our life we enjoy healthy brain function because our body is able to keep free-radical activity under control by manufacturing its own antioxidants from the proteins we eat. As aging takes place, the ability of our body to keep up the level of antioxidants needed declines, and so progressive oxidative damage can take place.

These are just two of the detrimental activities influencing mental acuity, memory functions, and sometimes depression associated with the aging process. However, they are two very important ones and, fortunately, those which can be beneficially influenced by dietary intervention.

How the Sea Can Help Maintain Mental Acuity and Brain Health

Many years ago it was a common theme that eating fish was beneficial for the brain, and that a healthy fish diet led to increased intelligence. However, the theme was based purely on observation and anecdotal information since the science was not understood. Advances in analytical procedures and knowledge of some of the mechanisms of the brain have now allowed us to have a much better understanding of the reason why this theme was soundly based.

For the brain to be healthy and function efficiently, it needs to have an adequate supply of the correct fuels. As we have seen earlier, many of these fuels can be manufactured by the body itself from compounds derived from standard nutrition. However, some fuels cannot be manufactured within the body and need to be provided by diet. In addition, the ability to manufacture some of the fuels can decline as we age. Some fuels are vital for efficient brain development even before a child is born and continue to be crucial throughout the lifetime. These fuels are the special long-chain fatty acids (commonly referred to as omega-3 or n-3 fatty acids), and the sea is the best source of these for dietary use. These fatty acids, in particular docosohexaenoic acid (DHA), are required for maintaining the flexibility and fluidity of the brain cell membranes, an important brain characteristic since it enhances the ability of the cells to transmit signals by flexing and contracting. In fact, DHA is the most abundant of the fats utilized in our brains.

It is also very important to have the appropriate ratio of the omega-3 fatty acids to the omega-6 fatty acids that are derived from meat and dairy products. The modern diet tends to imbalance this ratio in favor of the omega-6 fatty acids. Instead of a healthy ratio of about 1:1 (omega 3 to omega 6), it has become as high as 1:10 or even 1:20! Note how the theme of balance is evident yet again.

To provide an adequate supply of the long-chain (marine) fatty acids necessitates consumption of plenty of fish, particularly oily fish from cold seawater such as salmon, sardines, mackerel, and kahawai. Interestingly, including plenty of fish in the diet will also provide the important protein source for the specific amino acids needed for our neurotransmitters.

It is not always a simple matter for some people to have a regular diet of fish, and in this case the fuels for the brain can be obtained in a convenient form as nutritional supplements. Capsules of high-quality fish oils, having a high ratio of docoso-hexaenoic acid (DHA) to eicosapentaenoic acid (EPA), will provide the fatty acids to help restore the omega-3 to omega-6 balance as well as brain cell membrane fluidity. Because there are so many fish-oil products available, it will be advisable to check the label to establish the source and the relative levels of DHA and EPA. The fish-oil capsules alone will not, however, provide the marine proteins. A more comprehensive nutritional supplement that would supply the fatty acids for cell membrane health, the amino acids (from proteins) for neurotransmitter health, and even the antioxidant to reduce free-radical damage would contain a shellfish extract and a special fish oil. The shellfish extract could be the green-lipped mussel described in Chapter 3 because it contains the amino acids phenylalanine and tyrosine, plus the long-chain fatty acids, and a natural balanced content of minerals. The fish oil could be one with the suitable level of omega-3 fatty acids blended with squalene. Squalene is a marine hydrocarbon with excellent antioxidant activity to reduce free-radical damage and also good oxygen-carrying capacity to help maintain healthy brain cell metabolism. Here again, natural products derived from our planet's largest balanced medium, the seas, can help us maintain the balance of our mental medium, the brain.

10

OSTEOPOROSIS

In very general terms, osteoporosis is a disease in which our bone structure is weakened due to an inadequate content of calcium phosphate. It is a serious condition that, together with associated reduced bone density, affects up to 50 percent of postmenopausal women and 20 percent of men over the age of 50. It is therefore regarded as a major public health risk that, unfortunately, is exacerbated by some of our modern living habits such as lack of exercise, smoking, and alcohol consumption.

Our bones are formed from *collagen*, a protein that provides elasticity and flexibility, and *calcium phosphate*, a mineral salt that provides strength and rigidity. In a similar manner to the homeostasis situation in our joints (explained in Chapter 3), there is also a natural changeover of new bone for old. The parathyroid gland controls the blood levels of calcium, regulating the amount being removed from our bones to maintain blood levels in conjunction with dietary supplementation. This control is vital to prevent premature osteoporosis, elevated blood levels, and kidney damage. Up to the age of about 30 the rate of formation of new bone matches the resorption (loss) of old bone so that the system is nicely in balance. After this age, the rate of loss tends to exceed the rate of formation, creating a porosity in our bones with consequential structural weakening.

Certain dietary components and some medications are known to further the development of osteoporosis through their influence on calcium absorption and excretion. For example, red meats and some carbohydrates that contain high levels of phosphorous can inhibit the absorption of the soluble calcium phosphate salt. Fatty foods can also have an adverse effect on absorption of dietary calcium by creating insoluble calcium compounds that precipitate. On the other hand, foods such as salmon (eaten with the bones), dairy products, green leaf vegetables, and almonds each provide a good source of calcium.

Some medications, for example long-term use of corticosteroids prescribed in the treatment of arthritis, can lead to significant loss of bone density due to the double-barreled effect of reducing calcium absorption and increasing calcium excretion.

It is therefore apparent that, in order to minimize the adverse effects of osteoporosis and reduced bone density, our bodies need a regular supply of calcium in a form that is both easily digested and absorbed. The recommended amount of supplemental ionic calcium required each day ranges from 1000 to 1500 mg. Some of this will come from the normal diet of vegetables and dairy products. However, if it is to be derived from a supplemental source, the actual amount of calcium present in the supplement will be less than the total amount of supplement ingredient. For example, calcium products based on calcium carbonate will only yield 40 percent of the weight as calcium ion, the rest being carbonate ion.

As it happens, calcium is one of the most used minerals in our bodies and, together with other minerals and trace elements, it is responsible for a multitude of functions ranging from bone and teeth structure to control of muscle contraction and relaxation, brain cell impulses, and pH (acid/alkaline) balance. Of the calcium in our bodies, 99 percent is contained in our bones and teeth. However, the remaining 1 percent, which is contained in our body fluids, is responsible for all the other functions, including those mentioned above, an indication that it is not always a large amount of substance that is necessary to influence physiological body functions.

To be effective calcium needs to be in what is called its ionic state so that it is able to combine with other substances in the body. The digestive process will normally provide calcium in its ionic form, but the efficiency of this process and the yield of ionic calcium are influenced by the form in which the dietary calcium is consumed. For the calcium ions to be absorbed from the small intestine, it is important that an adequate supply of vitamin D is available. Without vitamin D, calcium will not be absorbed but will simply pass straight through the body. The absence of vitamin D plays a major role in causing Rickets, a disorder in very young children in which the bones remain soft due to inadequate calcium absorption. Vitamin D is naturally biosynthesized by the body in the presence of sunlight on the skin. In the absence of adequate sunlight, supplementation with vitamin D is essential.

The Sea in the Prevention of Osteoporosis

Supplementary calcium is available from a variety of sources such as proprietary formulations based on calcium carbonate, dairy products, and powdered oyster shell.

Dried and powdered *oyster shell* has been used for many years as a supplementary source of calcium and has the advantage over many other supplementary sources of a limited content of other minerals due to its origin in mineral-rich seawater. The absorption of ionic calcium from oyster-shell powder, however, is no better than that from good dairy sources, and it is *absorption* that is the important factor.

A product reported to have the highest absorption rate is, however, another product of the seas—*coral calcium*. Unfortunately, there are some extravagant and unsubstantiated claims being made for coral calcium, depicting it as a panacea for almost any illness. Its use in calcium supplementation for the inhibition of bone-density loss and osteoporosis is, nevertheless, valid. Corals are animals that mainly inhabit reefs, sometimes actually forming the reefs. They surround themselves with a strong-walled structure based on calcium salts. Their normal food is plankton, which they entrap with tentacles or sticky substances, depending on the species. It is the rigid wall structure of the corals that provides coral calcium. In addition to the fact that coral calcium is possibly the most easily digested and assimilated form of calcium (about 70 percent being bioavailable), its origin in the sea provides it with a wealth of other mineral components. Calcium absorption by the body, and its subsequent metabolism, are aided by the presence of other minerals. The fact that this product of the seas naturally contains the minerals necessary to aid its utilization by the body makes it a valuable choice for calcium supplementation.

It is also interesting to note that coral calcium can be used in reconstructive surgery where bone grafts are required. It appears that this form of calcium binds to the existing bone extremely well and grows into the existing bone to form a strong matrix with minimal rejection. Just another example of the potential of the seas to provide products that are highly compatible with the human body.

Note: If the harvesting of large amounts of coral calcium is not carefully controlled, it may pose a threat to the natural marine environment. Hopefully, careful management and regulation of the harvesting should allow successful regeneration to take place so that a sustainable resource is available.

11

RADIATION SICKNESS, THE THYROID, AND GOITER

L inking these disorders together in one chapter may at first appear strange. However, there is a common thread—the treatment for all three is contained in one marine product!

Radiation Sickness

Radiation sickness can take many forms, including the exacerbation of existing disease states, and also differs in intensity depending on the degree of exposure to low or high levels of radiation. It is important to recognize that it is not just atomic explosions that create radiation hazards. Diagnostic X-rays, TV screens, and other apparently noninvasive sources need to be considered. It is beyond the scope of this book to explore the complexity of radiation sickness or the range of treatments available to treat the condition. However, one particular treatment should be addressed here because it is a product of the seas. This is the common seaweed known as *kelp*.

Kelp has been shown to be effective in lowering strontium 90 and other radio isotope levels in laboratory animals and human beings subjected to radiation (Clark, L.). Scientists have also proven the beneficial effect that kelp has in lowering radioactive iodine levels in human patients. Although this can also be achieved by using elemental iodine, this is a relatively difficult procedure requiring medical supervision. If kelp is used instead, the natural iodine content of the seaweed performs the same function quite safely.

There are, however, more benefits to be gained by using kelp for lowering radio isotope levels in people. These are due to the natural content of a wide range of minerals in addition to sodium alginate and iodine. Some scientists have suggested that the mineral content of kelp may have a significant influence on its ability to reduce radioisotope levels in the body (Clark, L.). A very important point that has come out of the experimental use of seaweed for removing radioisotopes from humans is that the seaweed has lowered the level in bones as well as in the blood and other organs (Tanaka et al.). This natural product of the sea, which can reduce the level of a range of radioactive isotope levels in all the areas of the body without the complication of adverse side effects, is a good example of the power of natural marine products to treat even the diseases created by modern technology.

Thyroid and Goiter

The thyroid gland, which is situated in the front of the neck, is responsible for the production of hormones that perform a number of important functions in our bodies and are essential for life. The thyroid gland is, in turn, influenced by two other vitally important glands, the pituitary and the hypothalamus. These glands tend to control the hormone production and releasing functions of the thyroid by detecting high or low levels of thyroid hormones in the blood and producing hormones themselves that stimulate the thyroid into action. The two main problems associated with thyroid function are hypothyroidism and hyperthyroidism. In *hypothyroidism* the gland is producing too little thyroid hormone and in *hyperthyroidism* it is producing an excess of thyroid hormone.

Goiter is the name given to a condition in which the thyroid gland grows and causes swelling at the front of the neck due to the abnormal production of thyroid cells. This occurs because the pituitary gland is producing a hormone that helps the thyroid gland capture as much iodine from the food and water as possible. A secondary function of this hormone is causing the growth of thyroid cells. It is not difficult to understand that goiter is likely to be associated with areas where there is a natural iodine deficiency in the water, and there are many such areas around the world. The disease is more prevalent in females than males, possibly due to greater hormonal activity in females. There is another form of goiter, however, that is not directly associated with iodine deficiency but is due to the activity of a specific antibody that stimulates the production of excessive amounts of thyroid hormones. Careful diagnosis of the specific type of thyroid disease affecting a person is very important because treatment for one type may be aggravating to another.

Thyroid disorders are quite common in populations even where iodine deficiency is not a problem. In these cases it is usually a problem caused by autoimmune reactions in which abnormal antibodies (protein molecules programmed to recognize foreign invaders and act as our defense force) actually attack our own cells. In this case they attack the thyroid gland, causing it to stimulate the production of too much thyroid hormone (hyperthyroidism).

Scientists investigating potential causes for goiter and other thyroid disorders have established a link between hard drinking water containing fluoride and the incidence of the diseases. Where hard, fluoride-containing drinking water is present, there tends to be a higher incidence of the endemic type of goiter (this is the most common type linked to iodine deficiency) than in areas with soft water and lower fluoride levels. It is not really known if the effect of hard water and high fluoride reflects a total of the combined effect of both or just an enhanced effect of one due to the presence of the other. The possible function of fluoride in this respect is interesting, however, because chemically fluorine is allied to iodine and could have been thought to have a similar influence.

How the Sea Can Help Treat Goiter

For many years people with iodine deficiency have used tablets made from the kelp variety of seaweeds. These seaweeds are relatively rich in iodine, deriving it from the seawater in which they live. They are also rich in minerals and B-group vitamins, providing a nicely balanced mineral supplement to the body in a form that is easily assimilated. However, it is the iodine content that has been the important component for people suffering from goiter, the other valuable components simply being a bonus. Iodine naturally present in kelp tablets is reported to be more slowly assimilated than that in iodine solutions thus reducing the likelihood of allergic reactions. The use of iodized salts, which can be natural sea salts, is also a recognized method of adding iodine to the diet, and because these salts will be consumed in relatively small amounts at any one time, they are unlikely to cause ill effects.

Thyroid hormone production is a finely controlled function, operating to maintain the appropriate balance of these hormones in the blood. It is important to be sure that adding iodine to the diet is appropriate for the type of thyroid problem a person suffers from, and the advice of a doctor is recommended before kelp or any other iodine supplement is used. If iodine supplementation is recommended, then kelp, an herbal product of the sea, may be the best source.

12

FARMING THE SEAS FOR MEDICINES

I mentioned earlier in the book that I believe the farming of the New Zealand green-lipped mussel to produce a product used for the treatment of arthritis represents the first time in history that the seas were actively farmed on a large scale to produce a medicine. However, with the discovery of more natural medicinal products in a range of marine animals and plants, it will become increasingly important to develop methods of cultivation for these animals and plants. There are two fundamental reasons for this. One is that demand for treatments for some diseases, cancer being a good example, is likely to be so large that simply harvesting the natural resources to provide the medicinal product could damage the ecological balance in the seas with potentially devastating results. The other is that the production of medicinal products requires a reliable source of raw material to be available on a regular basis, and the raw material should be of a reasonably consistent quality. Usually this can only be achieved by using controlled cultivation procedures.

Some medicinal products will still have to be derived from animal species that are not suitable for farming, either because it is impractical to farm them on a sufficiently large scale or the farming of them is simply too difficult. An example of the problem of scale is farming cod for the supply of cod liver oil, and an example of being too difficult (not impossible, but grossly uneconomic) is farming deep sea dogfish for the provision of immunity-enhancing liver oil. Fortunately, in these cases and others like them, ecological damage or unreliable quality problems do not exist because the medicinal product is often derived as a by-product of normal harvesting and processing of food. Management quotas to ensure the sustainability of commercial fisheries are now in place for many species. Utilizing the by-products of a controlled industry—sometimes previously discarded as wastes—to produce valuable medicinal products is therefore a more efficient use of resources.

How Can the Seas Be Farmed?

In most instances farming the sea merely involves using the natural properties of seawater to grow a desired species of animal or plant under controlled conditions. The beauty of this is that no fertilizers, bactericides, or herbicides are used in the process. It is simply a case of designing the culture system so that the best environment for the species concerned, and the maximum value of the seawater for that species, are captured. Of course there can be the occasional exception to this situation, and the farming of salmon is an example. In this case the seawater enclosure is merely a suitable medium for the salmon to live in. They are fed artificial foods and, if shore tank cultivation is involved, they may even have some bactericidal components added to the tank water.

However, many species of both animals and plants are currently being farmed successfully without the need for any artificial assistance other than a substrate for them to attach to. The substrate can be completely inert so that it does not lend any nutritional or contaminating contribution to the environment. It is present to provide a controllable and, in certain cases, harvestable structure for the species being cultivated. For example, oysters are normally seeded as juveniles onto horizontal wooden racks or trays supported by vertical wooden posts. The farms are situated where the oysters will have the maximum time of coverage by seawater each tide, but will also be out of the water for a short period during each tide. There are some exceptions to this method where the oysters are cultivated on permanently submerged lines or structures, but there is a good reason why the first method is preferred. When oysters set naturally (not all species, but the ones normally cultivated), they normally set in areas of the shore between the high and low water marks. We may wonder why they do so, since the longer they are under water the more food they could eat. The answer is only known to the oyster. However, it is speculated that they need to spend some time in the air so that predatory organisms, which cannot survive out of the water, will not be able to develop on the oyster and harm it or perhaps simply compete for food by taking up residence on its shell. This is an example of nature exerting a subtle influence that man has had to copy, since the logical approach would have suggested that permanent immersion would be better.

Mussels, on the other hand, benefit by being immersed in the sea continuously. Mussels are normally cultivated by attaching the seed (baby) mussels to ropes that are then suspended vertically in the sea, allowing the shellfish to benefit from the total water column. Spanish mussel farmers tend to use moored rafts from which they suspend ropes, whereas New Zealanders (and others) usually run long lines along the sea surface, supported by floats. The vertical ropes hang down at regular intervals from these surface lines. Like oysters, mussels are filter-feeders; therefore the more seawater, containing the planktonic food they require and are able to filter, the better they grow. There is, however, another significant advantage in having the mussels attached to ropes suspended vertically as opposed to having them laid on the seabed. This is freedom from one of their main enemies, the starfish. Starfish are able to rapidly devastate a bed of mussels if they have access to it. The starfish will wrap itself around the mussel, attach the suction pads on its arms to each shell, and exert a constant pressure against the powerful closure muscles of the shellfish. Gradually the muscles holding the shellfish closed will weaken and the starfish will then extend its stomach into the shellfish and digest it. Starfish are extremely hardy animals; they can survive even after losing several arms (they just grow replacements!) and represent a serious threat to mussel populations. Fortunately, they do not swim up from the seabed, so mussels on the vertical ropes are safe.

Some seaweeds are now cultivated on marine farms as well as being harvested naturally from feral beds, such as the kelp beds off the California coast. Farming of these is usually achieved by having the juvenile plants or cuttings attached to ropes that are suspended vertically or horizontally in the sea. While this method is not suitable for cultivating the huge kelps because they are more suited to a stable seabed environment where they can anchor themselves firmly, it does lend itself to some of the smaller algae such as Undaria and Nori. Because these algae do not feed through a root system (the roots are normally just for securing themselves to a substrate), they merely require light and access to nutrients in the seawater for growth to occur.

In the chapter on cancer treatments from the sea, it was mentioned that the marine sponges are probably the most prolific source of biologically active compounds with the potential to treat cancers. While synthesis of the active compounds discovered in the sponges may become economically viable, it does not automatically follow that they will be as effective as the naturally produced compound, or as available for general use because of the high cost of synthetic processing. Therefore sponge farming is desirable and, fortunately, in many cases it is quite possible. By appearance, the marine sponges are very unsophisticated and completely sedentary in their lifestyle. It is difficult to see how they survive because, like all biological beings, they have to eat, reproduce, and, in their environment in particular, protect themselves against predators. It is the very basic biological structuring to accomplish these functions that provides them with the highly potent, complex chemical components that we have discovered can be so valuable for treating our diseases.

Sponges can be cultivated, and currently some are being cultivated on marine farms. These farms simply require areas of the seabed that are suitable for attaching pieces of sponge to a solid substrate, such as stones, and that have the right combination of temperature, light, and natural nutritional characteristics. Because they are permanently submerged and not really appropriate for operating by dredging, these farms are usually worked using divers. However, if the demand for a supply of naturally produced sponge compounds increases, the scale of sponge farming will also increase and this will lead to the development of alternative methods for larger-scale operations.

Already being experimented with, and almost certain to become a feature of future marine farming processes, is *polyculture.* This involves designing and placing the marine farm so that a diversity of species can be cultivated on one site. Initially this is more readily achieved in land farms employing seawater tank systems, but it need not be restricted to this. The critical requirements for polyculture are that each species on the farm has different nutritional demands and, in some cases, can tolerate water conditions that have been modified by the species preceding it in the farm system. In the future it may be possible to utilize the benefits of symbiosis for some types of polyculture. *Symbiosis* describes the situation where organisms live together in harmony because each depends on the other for growth and survival.

Another area of marine farming that could be utilized is a type of polyculture in which animals grown for one purpose will supply product for an entirely different purpose. Examples of this are abalone and oyster farming specifically to produce pearls. However, the meat from both of these animals can be used for food and, in the case of the oyster in particular, can also provide a product with therapeutic properties. In New Zealand, closed-circuit seawater tank farms are now being used for the cultivation of abalone pearls (the New Zealand species of abalone is called Paua), with the flesh being a highly regarded delicacy.

In the future we will see farms developed for the cultivation of seahorses because, apart from a growing demand for these animals for culinary purposes in Asian countries, they contain a substance that can be beneficial in the treatment of urinary incontinence. Harvesting of these attractive creatures from the wild will not sustain market growth for either of these purposes without endangering the natural ecology, and farm cultivation will therefore be necessary.

In this chapter we have looked at just a few examples of farming the seas for the production of medicinal products. Because so much of our planet's biological productivity is in the seas and the diversity of species is so great, it is obvious that, in the years ahead, more species with valuable natural therapeutic components will be discovered and methods of cultivation for these will need to be developed. A very important factor to be taken into consideration for such development will be the environmental impact of the farming processes.

Environmental Factors in Marine Farming

The term *environmental factors* covers a wide range of topics. These embrace environmental impacts that, on the one hand, might adversely affect the farming process and, on the other hand, might adversely affect the local ecology or even aesthetic value and public enjoyment of an area. Factors that could adversely affect marine farming would include changes to land use adjacent to the farm site, shore-based developments that increased the level of rainwater runoff into rivers or streams flowing into farmed areas, man-made constructions that change tidal flow patterns, and pollution.

In considering why these would adversely influence farming of the seas, we have to remember that this activity takes place in relatively shallow waters close to the land. The reason for this is that marine farms that are not shore-based require sheltered water conditions with reasonably simple access. However, the shore-based farms can be similarly influenced because they draw their seawater supply from the area close to the land-based site. Deep, offshore waters are generally unsuitable for marine farms because they present difficulties for anchoring and can be too violent both for the animals being cultivated and the means of tending them on a regular basis.

We might question how the change of land use on the shore adjacent to a marine farm site might influence the farm adversely. An example of this could be the clearing of land for use in agriculture in which crop spraying is necessary. Runoff from the land during rain could carry contaminants into the farm area. Shore-based developments, such as new housing or industrial estates, can have a significant influence on estuarine and close coastal waters. The increased runoff of rainwater due to the existence of roof areas, use of hoses for washing cars, as well as other activities carries garden sprays, oils, and other road-surface contaminants with it into stormwater drains, ending up in streams and rivers that drain into the sea. These may then flow right through a farm area and contaminate the crop. Note that I have referred to changes in land use in discussing these factors. Obviously, a farm would not be placed in an area where this situation already existed.

The word pollution covers a multitude of possibilities. For example, perfectly clean drinking water is a pollutant in the sea! If sufficient pure rainwater flows into an estuary or shallow coastal area it can dilute the natural salt content of the seawater to a level that is not tolerable for many of the natural inhabitants. While some animals, salmon and flounder being examples, can tolerate water that is salt or fresh, most will die if transferred from one to the other because osmosis causes the loss of critical body-fluid components. Possibly more insidious forms of pollution, however, are those that do not affect the species being farmed but which do affect the person eating the farmed animal or being treated with a product derived from the animal. This form of pollution can be carried through several steps in the food chain, perhaps starting off in food eaten by plankton, passing into the organism eating the plankton, and so on up the chain to the final consumer. Common examples of these contaminating organisms belong to a group of planktonic algae known as dinoflagellates. They contain compounds that can cause a variety of toxic effects in people, ranging from diarrhea through amnesia to paralysis. For example paralytic shellfish poisoning is caused by a toxin called saxitoxin, which is present in the Gonyaulax species of dinoflagellates. Another toxin, responsible for neurotoxic shellfish poisoning, is brevetoxin from the dinoflagellate *Gymnodinium breve*. The degree of toxicity is related to the concentration of the dinoflagellate in the water, and thus in the host animal. Fortunately, these contaminants are known and can be detected in routine quality-control assays. Constant vigilance is necessary however, and sophisticated monitoring procedures have now been established for the detection of possible biotoxin contaminants that can infect shellfish farms and cause problems for human consumers of the products. Realizing this, it is obvious that any shellfish or shellfish derivatives intended for human or animal consumption must only come from areas that are carefully and routinely monitored.

These contaminants are an example of an indirect effect of pollution. They come from algae that the shellfish consume as part of their natural filter-feeding process but do not affect the shellfish itself. However, the algae that carry these contaminants need a healthy supply of nutrients in order to grow to an effective level. A combination of the nutrients derived from sewage plus sunlight serves the algae well in this respect. We therefore introduce the indirect influence of sewage pollution, not necessarily affecting the farmed species, but providing the nutrients for the development of another organism that does affect it.

Of course, domestic sewage can be detrimental to marine farming, but this is dependent to a degree on the length of time the sewage is in the water before reaching the farm area and the nature of the sewage. Bacterial contaminants may not be a problem because the natural antibiotic effect of seawater will destroy them quite quickly. Viruses however are a different matter, and some can survive for a considerable time even in cold seawater. Other contaminants such as oils and detergents can also have damaging effects, and marine farms would not normally be placed in an area that might be subject to sewage pollution. This having been said, we sometimes forget that it is not only humans who produce fecal pollution. Farm animals and birds also contribute, and the effect of contamination by seabirds must be taken into consideration. Fortunately, fecal contamination is easy to check and is normally a standard part of the quality-control procedure whether a product is destined for food or medicine.

Finally, we might consider how man-made structures could influence a marine farm. When a site for a marine farm is chosen, the selection is based on adequate depth, accessibility, mooring requirements, and water flow. The last parameter will be crucial to the productivity of the farm since it will influence the amount of food available for the species being cultivated. The building of new structures (wharves, groynes, training walls, etc.) that change the flow of the water through the farm could significantly reduce the amount of food available and hence the viability of the farm.

In discussing some of these environmental influences that might impact on farming the seas for medicine, we also need to consider the impact that farming the seas for medicine might have on the environment.

By placing a marine farm in an area of the sea that was previously just open water, we will create an ecological impact on that area. This impact will be in the form of a higher density of population of a particular species than would normally inhabit that area and a possible adverse ecological impact resulting from the presence of this species. The adverse ecological impact could be smothering of benthic (bottom-dwelling) organisms beneath the farm or lack of food for other indigenous organisms due to competition from the farmed species. There could also be over-settlement of juveniles from the farmed species, resulting in the displacement of other indigenous inhabitants. All of these factors should be, and normally are, taken into account when applications for a license to farm an area of the sea are being considered. A considerable amount of data for use in a variety of different situations has been established by long-term scientific research.

More work still needs to be done, however, due to the complex nature of the sea as a farming medium and the biology of many of the marine animals and plants.

Apart from the ecological impacts of marine farms, there are aesthetic and navigational impacts to be considered. People who have built homes with beautiful sea views do not normally want to see rows of buoys or floats as part of their outlook. Boating enthusiasts want to have freedom to sail in coastal waters without the hindrance of marine farm structures. Here again it is important that these factors are considered at the application stage for the farms because neither of these impacts need be a problem if properly addressed. Some marine farms are already being changed so that the flotation units supporting the top of the farm are under the surface. Although it is essential that the boundaries of the farm, usually only the four corners, are clearly marked with surface buoys for the safety of navigation, the visual impact is significantly reduced. In other cases, judicious place-ment of farms can avoid any aesthetic impact problems entirely. There are valid arguments for and against the navigational impact. Those who argue that these farms restrict navigation claim the hazard of ropes and buoys reducing the area for free navigation, while others argue that the regulatory lights required to mark marine farms provide added navigational aids at night in areas where there was total darkness. There have also been instances where lives have been saved by the presence of a marine farm because people were able to climb onto farm structures or hold onto buoys when they were in the water after an accident. Properly situated and marked, there is no reason for marine farms to present a hazard to navigation by competent sailors.

As mentioned earlier, cultivating a particular species of ani-mal or plant is bound to have some influence on the ecology of the area supporting the marine farm. However, the influence need not be adverse and, in many cases can be beneficial, even though it is changing the natural ecology. One such scenario is where the farm is situated in an area that, due to the nature of the tidal flows, does not have a natural settlement of the species being farmed but, as a result of the farm's presence, a settlement occurs. Experience with large-scale shellfish farming has indicated that nature's natural selection process will normally limit any such effect to a balanced level. Were this not the case, the competitive demand for food would be disadvantageous for the farms. Another example of a beneficial environmental impact from shellfish cultivation is enhanced fish populations surrounding the farms. Not only has this been good for the fish, but also for human anglers who have experienced excellent fishing in the proximity of shellfish farms.

Overall, considering the enormous benefit that can be provided for people suffering serious and debilitating diseases by marine farms that cultivate animals or plants containing natural therapeutic substances, farming the seas for medicines makes a highly desirable and valuable contribution to our future health and well-being.

13

PERSONAL EXPERIENCES

The inclusion of personal testimonials in books dealing with medicinal products is often heavily criticized because the information, classed as subjective rather than objective (as is the case in controlled studies), is deemed unreliable. However, the point can and should be made that the information (provided that it is unsolicited) is being given by *experts* in the disease because they are actually suffering from it! In the case of arthritic disorders, it would be highly unlikely for someone to write a glowing account of how he or she has been helped by a product if this were not definitely so. While, in some instances, there is the possibility of natural remission having coincided with the use of the product, this would be a rare occurrence, and the same factor would apply equally to any other therapy.

The following personal accounts are all genuine extractions from letters or verbal reports sent, or given, either to me personally or to the company that produces the marine substances referred to. I make no apology for their inclusion, but have omitted the trade name of the products. Personal accounts relating to only two of the diseases described in this book have been included in this chapter. However, they are the diseases most frequently experienced worldwide. The letters are considered to be representative of the sort of results that can be achieved with quality and well-researched natural marine products, and they are printed here in the hope that they may give encouragement to others. I firmly believe that, provided it is based on genuine facts, encouragement leading to a positive attitude to recovery from disease is in itself a valuable therapy.

While the names of the writers have been omitted for reasons of privacy, all have readily given permission for their letters to be used. The letters or excerpts are printed as written, even if they are not grammatically correct. Accounts similar to those printed here have been received in several languages other than English because the diseases involved have no international boundaries. Translation of these accounts has revealed the same sentiments being expressed.

Most of the personal accounts recorded here relate to arthritis, and there are several reasons for this. Possibly the main reason is that so many people and animals experience this disorder that correspondence from just a small percentage of these would represent a huge number. However, there is no doubt in my mind that most of the people have written because their relief from pain and disability, without the worry of other problems being caused by the treatment, has prompted them to share their beneficial experiences with others suffering similar conditions.

Arthritis

In some of the correspondence received, a significant amount of helpful detail has been presented. An example of this is indicated in the following two excerpts.

> Further to our telephone conversation in May last, I can now advise you further of my progress with a little more confidence than I had at the time. You will recall that I was

suffering a 'flare-up' and although it was a nuisance I know enough now not to get too despondent.

I therefore continued with five capsules a day of Green-Lipped Mussel Extract and gritted my teeth! From a purely clinical approach I think the best I can do is itemize the pattern of things as they stand at present.

1. The latest flare-up from inception to completion has lasted approximately two months. It commenced noticeably about the beginning of May last. I had unusual stress at the time with family problems too.
2. Since roughly a week ago (3rd. July) the pain has dramatically eased. At first I thought that it was wishful thinking and could not have abated. (I always think this when it seems too good to be true!) However, I have now been moving around with greater comfort continually for a week and therefore feel confident to announce publicly that I have reached another stage of healing.
3. Once again my leg has the sensation of being longer— although I realize it is obviously the muscles getting stronger and therefore regaining their natural shape and size after their wastage.
4. Because the leg appears more elastic I do not have terrible pulling and burning pain in my right buttock, back and indeed the whole of the trunk of my body. I appeared at one time to have lost the whole muscle power four-dimensional, i.e., length, front, back and side!

Measured against the state I was in a year ago, it is a joy not to continually tremble, especially in the trunk of my body— absolutely no control over the nerves it would seem at the time. So—from this standpoint—a very great measure of improvement in strength.

5. Still a marked presence of ammonia in body wastage at the end of the day.
6. When I stand I am able to have both knees nearly level as opposed to having to bend the 'good leg' to accommodate the affected leg approximately 5". I am able to walk in the fashion of heel-toe now without distress, instead of walking on my toes on that foot because the

back of the leg just could not stretch down. The whole leg appears more flexible.

7. My conclusion is that when I suffer pain, it is a good sign because when it clears my leg has certainly been getting back to normal in all ways. The calf muscles have regained their proper shape and it is not so obvious that they are wasted when measured against the good leg.

8. I am able to walk a short way indoors without the aid of a walking stick and without falling heavily over to one side each time I place my foot on the ground. The footsteps I have been taking in the last couple of days have been normally balanced and most important of all, there has been no pain, not even a feeling of soreness in the joints when I have placed my foot on the ground.

9. I do not intend to try walking outdoors without the aid of the walking stick until nature shows me without doubt that all is back to normal. I intend to continue to take 5 capsules a day until I am walking without the stick and still without pain—perhaps to the extent of taking a whole bottleful before the next step. I then propose to drop my daily intake to four capsules per day for maybe a full bottle, then three capsules for a full bottle.

I think that if I can get to the happy stage of no pain and back to normal I shall, for as long as the extract is produced, continue to take one capsule a day for the rest of my life.

10. The whole limb appears to have been lubricated because I cannot remember now the sickening noise resembling castanets or dry twigs breaking when I endeavored to bend the limb. I have been taking the Green-Lipped Mussel Extract at full prescribed dosage continually since the commencement of last August, therefore it is the best part of a year now, and when deliberately comparing my strength to this time last year it is astonishing how near I am to being normal again!

The benefit that this person has received by taking the mussel extract is evident from the amount of detail included in the letter. It is also obvious that this person was seriously incapacitated and yet the product has had such a significant effect on the condition.

Another example of a very detailed letter comes from a gentleman in Spain. It reads:

To conclude this year I feel obliged to inform you about my miraculous experience with Green-Lipped Mussel Extract. I already told you something of my background in my first letter and that I badly suffered with rheumatoid poly-arthritis during the past months. From August on I have been treated here with all hard medical drugs of the pirarolones, butaphenaralone and corticosteroid groups without any lasting results. Sometimes a certain relief but upon ceasing with a specific medication after a few days from bad to worse again. I felt poisoned by medicines, lost my appetite and felt depressed. No wonder as I saw the wheelchair coming towards me. I stopped therefore all cures and felt a little better when the side effects disappeared. At that time the balance was: active arthritis in the right knee accompanied by a serious bursitis, active arthritis in right ankle joints, right thumb and indicator finger, left wrist and crippled four fingers, right shoulder and shoulder blade and also some pain in adjoining ribs.

On the 13th. December I started with Green-Lipped Mussel Extract. The first eight days, no change. On the ninth day increasing pain in all affected joints with slight fever till the thirteenth day (without fever and decreasing pain). On the fourteenth day all other joints which were affected in the preceding years showed symptoms of becoming active again accompanied by again slight fever.

On the fifteenth day, however, I awoke for the first time with hardly any arthritic pain although stiffness and immobility still remained. From the sixteenth to the twentieth everything improved gradually, which caused a feeling of well being. From the twenty-first to the twenty-third day another revival of arthritic pain and slight fever but now in all joints affected now and in former years. But on the twenty-fourth day this was all gone. From thereon a gradual decrease of muscle tensions, stiffness and a slowly increasing mobility in all affected joints. Swollen right knee and ankle slowly diminishing.

On the thirty-second day able to walk again. On the forty-second day mobility, apart from some trouble of joint deformations, nearly normal for my age, hardly any pain, pleasant mobility! I am able to use all affected joints again without pain and with only some slight limitations and I can now carry out again the usual odd jobs around the house. I can walk again without trouble although I have to be careful with the use of my right leg as both knee and ankle joints were rather badly damaged.

Six weeks ago I had to pass my days, as a still dynamic person, in bed or on a couch. A sad prospect! Incidentally I also noticed a beneficial side effect. Small cuts and grazes are now healing, as I estimate, about twice as quickly as before.

PS. My wife and I are sailing on the 10th of next month from Las Palmas on a world cruise which we desperately nearly had to cancel!

Although these two quoted excerpts are rather long, it is appropriate to include them because they confirm some of the points made earlier about the properties of the extract. They also indicate that people who are suffering as seriously as this are able to give a detailed and accurate account of the changes in their condition and are not likely to be easily influenced by quack remedies.

Fortunately not all cases are as severe as the two just quoted, but, to the person involved, their situation can be just as desperate.

A letter from a lady in Italy indicates the joy and relief that come from simply being able to lead a normal life without constant pain.

I begin to feel like an agent in Rome as so many people have remarked on my wonderful improvement and want to try Green-Lipped Mussel Extract themselves that I am constantly getting it for someone.

You will be pleased to hear that I count myself one of the very lucky ones—not only am I restored to mobility, I am free of a constant pain that was almost intolerable. I was taking painkilling drugs three times per day to alleviate the distress but since I finished my first course of Green-Lipped Mussel

Extract I have not needed to take them. I have been able to get into and out of a chair without help, and have even tried knitting again.

I took a second course, following on the first bottle, and now need the courage to stop taking them for a time to judge the long-term effects. The results for me are incredible and almost unbelievable. The best part is that I do not need any drugs whatever now. I have really gone quite mad and am doing all sorts of things which have been impossible for some time.

Though I have to admit to being tired and full of aches I still do not have that terrible pain. There is a huge difference in aches and real pain. I only hope that other people will benefit as I have done. I am truly grateful and tell anyone who wants to listen to me just what happened.

A very brief letter from Nigeria indicates that arthritis is not restricted to the cold climates of the world; it is a worldwide disorder.

You may be interested to learn that after one course of Green-Lipped Mussel Extract my wife, who has suffered from arthritis for years, is now without pain in her joints, can bend and stretch much more easily and can now clench her hands— all without pain and without any side effects. Marvelous.

A British seaman wrote from London:

I would like you to convey my sincere thanks to the staff that produce and market Green-Lipped Mussel Extract. If the staff realized how much pain the capsules prevented me having in the last few years they would be very proud of what they produce as once again I say thank you to one and all.

My first benefit from Green-Lipped Mussel Extract was an increase in my sleeping hours. Prior to taking them I was fortunate to get two hours sleep in a night. At the present time I can get six to eight hours sleep free from pain. If anyone mentions arthritis to me my first words to them are to go on a course of Green-Lipped Mussel Extract. I will keep on recommending your product because I would like to see others get the benefit as much as I have done from the capsules.

A brief letter from a sheep farmer's wife in New Zealand brings in a very interesting point in that the mussel extract can help with conditions such as ankylosing spondylitis.

> I would like you to know that your Green-Lipped Mussel Extract capsules are helping my husband who has ankylosing spondylitis of the neck, spine and hips (for over twenty years). He finds considerable relief in his back and is able to drench sheep in comfort. He is fifty-five and his stoop had been getting progressively worse over the years. I thought I would let you know of his benefit as you are in a position to advise others.

Apart from pain and the lack of mobility there are other factors connected with arthritic disorders which can cause distress, particularly where deformities are involved. The next two letters clearly demonstrate the relief felt by the writers when Green-Lipped Mussel Extract helped their condition.

> My joints are ugly and deformed, but still useable and able to carry on next day, even after hard work on the previous one.
>
> My new discovery is that, when restless in the early part of the night because of soreness and swelling and blotchiness in my fingers, if I take another capsule any time between midnight and 3 a.m. I am able within minutes to drop into a peaceful sleep and am unaware of the pain in my hands which look quite clear of blotches and slender when next I see them. They are white and active and ready to use in the morning. A most thrilling discovery and one I tell my friends about.

Sometimes information comes in letters from people suffering arthritic disorders that describes an effect on other conditions associated with the disease but for which we had no previous data. The next letter illustrates this point.

> I thought I would put pen to paper and let you know that I have been taking Green-Lipped Mussel Extract now for approximately nine years. At first I started taking it for my arthritis which was at that time affecting my hips and found

complete relief. However I also have dermatitis or eczema very bad since birth and many years had to be wrapped in bandages. As I grew older my skin always looked red and chapped so on taking the capsules I found my skin becoming not so bad or dry looking. I found this out after taking two bottles and then, not having any arthritis pain, stopped taking the capsules and after about a month my skin became red and itchy again. So now although I still get arthritis at times in various parts I take it all the time mainly for my skin. I thought I would write and tell you. It might help someone else.

There is a tendency to imagine that medical problems only affect the doctors' patients and never the doctors themselves! This is, of course, not true, and there have been many communications from doctors about the effect that Green-Lipped Mussel Extract has had in their particular case. Many of these were verbal communications and usually involved some technical questions. However, a report sent by letter from a physician in Canada is reproduced below.

I am over eighty years old and a physician with more than fifty years experience and can observe results with an objective judgement. My condition, spondylosis of the lumbar vertebrae, from which I have suffered for twenty years improved dramatically. I had tried many other treatments which did not help. My chronic rheumatism in both legs which made walking painful and slow, became so much better within only five days that I could walk again quite easily. I could hardly believe the result. After finishing the two bottles I tried to get them again but was only able to obtain a variety which contained an addition of Brewers Yeast, was darkish yellow and smelled of smoked fish. The improvement I had experienced gradually disappeared and the new capsules did not help at all.

The letter goes on to request a supply of the genuine McFarlane product, and it clearly demonstrates the danger of fake and imitation products trying to take advantage of a situation with no thought for the people suffering the disease!

Another person in the medical profession, who would also be well-trained in making objective assessments of results, writes:

I am writing in praise of your product Green-Lipped Mussel Extract. Nearly two years ago I developed rheumatoid arthritis of both wrists and spondylosis of the cervical spine. My doctor prescribed the usual anti-inflammatory drugs, but as a State Registered Nurse, and having seen the side effects of these drugs on patients I have nursed, I was naturally very reluctant to take the medication.

Leading a very busy life as a wife, mother and holding down a full time nursing job, I decided to try other things. I tried homeopathy which turned out to be very expensive, and for me, not all that successful. Then I read an article about the mussel extract. I toyed with the idea of trying it, then at the company where I work as the Occupational Health Nursing Sister, I talked to a young man who is a sufferer of polyarthritis (and has had a hip replacement operation). He told me that he had a book about the green-lipped mussel which he let me read. I was impressed and decided to try a course of the capsules. This was in April this year. The book said that some people had to take the capsules for several months before experiencing relief. I was prepared to persevere. I was pretty desperate at the time.

I was very unwell. Low in health and in spirit. Unable to sleep at night, loss of power in my arms, shoulders, wrists and hands. I considered I was in the prime of life (forty-nine) and had got ten years or so to go before retiring from my nursing job. I found that in the mornings I could hardly lift my arms to dress and comb my hair. The pain was excruciating but I would not be beaten and continued to go to work each day.

I took the maximum dose of Green-Lipped Mussel Extract daily. Very slowly I began to notice an improvement by the summer May/June. The heat and swelling began to ease in the wrists. Then some days the pain would return to its maximum, especially if I was overtired or had done certain household jobs but somehow I felt I could cope a little better.

By the time September arrived, I knew that I was at last getting true result. Restful nights, a feeling of well being, only the very occasional and mild ache in the neck, wrists, shoulders and muscles. In fact so slight to what I had been having that I could almost ignore the discomfort. Had I attempted to type a letter like this a few weeks ago I would have been in tremendous pain! I noticed that in the October's issue of my magazine *Nursing Mirror* that someone had written to the "Your Questions Answered" page stating that she and her husband had been taking the mussel extract for over a year and found them to be most beneficial. In fact it seems their results are very similar to my own.

This letter graphically describes the emotional and physical stages that some arthritis sufferers go through and the eventual joy when lasting relief is found.

Finally, the following letter is an example of the possible temporary exacerbation of pain, experienced by a small percentage of people.

About seven years ago I heard of Green-Lipped Mussel Extract and discussed it with my doctor who stated that it could do no harm and if I wanted to waste money to try it. I immediately asked the chemist for some and started the course. Immediately the joints became more painful and I could easily have thrown the tablets away but for my husband's powers of persuasion. Then, within about two months, I found I could walk short distances and was much more active. Six months later I took another course of treatment with still further improvement and decided to stop the butazone altogether. Since then I take a course of Green-Lipped Mussel capsules about every nine months and though I still have aches and pains while taking the capsules I find that after each course there is still more improvement in the things I can do.

There are so many letters like this, but it is not possible to print them all in this book. Some of the letters relate to young children with Still's disease, a form of arthritis affecting the very young. Others relate to the results with both pet and commercial animals. A few examples of such communications follow.

You sent me a bottle of Green-Lipped Mussel Extract Tablets three weeks ago for my fourteen-year-old cat about whom we were very worried because she was limping badly with arthritis.

The result of taking two tablets a day is almost unbelievable for she now gallops around our one-third of an acre garden. Yes it's true!

Also her coat is gleaming with health and she could, in my opinion, pass for a youthful four-year-old.

Large dogs, particularly Labradors and German Shepherds tend to be prone to arthritic problems in their later years. A touching letter from a New Zealand lady describes the benefit that the product afforded her dog and hence the happiness of her family.

I feel I must write to you what is perhaps my last letter in praise of Green-Lipped Mussel Extract. Chubby, our Labrador, was put to sleep at Christmas and you may remember that she was one of the early animals to try the mussel extract some four or five years ago. At that time she had arthritis in the spine and hind legs and the vet was unable to do anything for her. From being unable to walk even the length of our driveway, once on the mussel extract she gradually progressed to become very agile, being able to leap up into the van, catch birds on the wing, etc. In fact she lived a normal, healthy and active life.

Last Christmas she was frisky one second and paralyzed the next—her spinal condition finally caught up with her.

However, I am positive that Green-Lipped Mussel Extract gave her and us five years of happy life which could not otherwise have been possible.

Another Labrador letter, this time from England.

I have recently come within an ace of having to make the sad decision to have my beloved Labrador/cross bitch, Bess, put down owing to the progress made by her condition of ankylosing spondylitis. At only the eighth day after taking three Green-Lipped Mussel Extract capsules a day she ceased to drag her right foot, ceased to walk (stagger rather) on the tops of her feet instead of the soles, due to loss of sensation, suffer less pain and begin to regain interest in life. In a fortnight she was once again able to walk far more steadily and her legs stopped splaying outward.

She has now recovered her ability to step up over stairs where she had to be carried and is now going out for walks again, albeit walking slowly.

She is thirteen (ninety-one by our age) so I think this is a remarkable result which I am sure will be progressive. Her coat has got a brand new gloss and I notice her eyes are fuller.

Letters have been received from the owners of all sorts of dogs, mostly pets, but some show dogs and breeding stock. The following letter is an example of one type of working dog.

My cocker spaniel is used for field-trialing and gamebird hunting in season and also rabbit and hare hunting so you can imagine he has an active life.

Last January he started breaking down with very little work and limping around quite badly. My veterinarian X-rayed him and could not be sure what the problem was but thought that he might be slipping a disc in his back or suffering from a rheumatic condition. He suggested complete rest as a possible cure. Resting him did not work so I decided to try the mussel extract at the beginning of April. He improved almost immediately and has now had a very full gamebird hunting season over the last eight weeks without any signs of breaking down and in fact is working faster than ever before.

Finally, just two examples of letters from horse owners. Most product use with horses is in racing and training stables. Communications from these has tended to be by telephone rather than letter; however, the sentiments and the stories of quite remarkable recoveries are the same.

The filly we are treating with your mussel extract has improved markedly after 3 months treatment. She was X-rayed in December 1979 when the vet stated that it was the worst case of arthritis and ring-bone he had seen that year. Butazolidine and Cortisone were given without effect—the filly's rump muscles wasted and some considered she should be destroyed as she became emaciated (it was a back leg which was affected).

As she was a thoroughbred filly and may have a value as a brood mare, not to mention sentimental value, we started feeding her the mussel extract. Now after three months she is fit, shining coat, well covered, her back muscles have regenerated and she walks, trots and gallops with very little sign of a limp. She was X-rayed again last month and it was found that ankylosis had taken place, the boney growths around the joint were smoothing and the joint generally had a tidier appearance.

This letter continues with more details about the filly and possibilities for her future. It is the excerpt above which is the important part for us.

The second example is a letter from the owner of a pacer in New Zealand.

You may recall that I obtained mussel extract from you some time ago to treat my pacer (name omitted). This horse was broken down with muscular trouble at the time.

Following treatment with the mussel extract (name omitted) was back on the track again and won four races before being sold to the USA.

Since being in the USA he has recorded times of under 2 minutes for the mile on several separate occasions. I thought that this information might be of interest to you and to others who may have a horse with arthritic or lameness problems.

The Common Cold, Influenza, and Viral Diseases

The first account below was not given to me but is my own firsthand experience with the use of deep sea shark liver oil for protection against colds and influenza.

I began to take 1000 mg per day of the deep sea shark liver oil described in Chapter Six about seven years ago and have continued to do so ever since. Despite often being in close proximity to people coughing and spluttering, (it is difficult not to be nowadays, particularly if traveling by air) I have not had to suffer the discomfort of either common cold or influenza for more than one day each time I have been infected. Leading a normal life, it is not practicable to protect against being infected but, if we have a strong immune system which immediately goes to war against the invading viruses, we need only suffer the one day while the battle rages and the invaders are wiped out. This has been my experience. I have felt the discomfort in my throat and back of my nose, which usually precedes the outbreak of a cold or influenza, then after about 24 hours of this have felt fine again. One of the best examples of my protective effect was when I traveled from New Zealand to Europe and back with a younger colleague who was not taking any antiviral prophylactic. We were together for most of the time and sat next to each other on flights. When we arrived home to New Zealand my colleague had to go straight home to bed with a hearty dose of influenza while I was able to go to work totally clear!

Two accounts from ladies in South Africa are of significant interest because they deal with conditions other than the common cold and influenza but which are related to the body's immune responses. Each of these ladies gave their account to me personally so that I could pass on their experience to others.

The first of these relates to the effect of the product on the immune response to allergy.

The lady told me that for eight years she had suffered with a most distressing condition in which she would have severe bouts of violent coughing at least three times every day. Each bout would last up to half an hour and when it eventually stopped she would be left exhausted and drained of energy. No treatment had been successful for her and she was very depressed. The physical aspect of the coughing fits was bad enough, but there was an emotional aspect also. She was unable to attend social functions or the theatre, because the coughing attacks tended to occur at such times and would create an intolerable disturbance. Even social functions at home proved difficult and stressful because once an attack began she would be unable to hold a conversation for up to thirty minutes and this was embarrassing for her guests.

Her condition appeared to be linked to some sort of immune dys-

function, having some similar characteristics to an allergy reaction, so she decided to try the deep sea shark liver oil product. After two months of consuming capsules providing 1000 mg daily the coughing bouts ceased completely. At the time of my meeting with her, one year since she started with the product, she had reduced to 500 mg daily as a maintenance course and had not suffered the coughing attacks again. Coincidentally she commented that she had also been free from colds during that year.

The other account concerns the young son of a lady who spoke with me and relates the effect of deep sea shark liver oil on a specific type of allergic response, asthma.

The lady told me that her son, now aged twelve years, had suffered since being a young baby from asthma. Seven months prior to my meeting with her she had started the boy on the deep sea shark liver oil capsules at 500 mg per day. She was both surprised and delighted to tell me that the symptoms began to improve and the characteristic wheezing and coughing gradually disappeared. At the time of our meeting, the asthma attacks had ceased. A side benefit of this dramatic change in the boy's health and breathing was that he had been accepted to a prestigious school and enrolled in the school choir. The boy was now continuing to take a daily maintenance course of the capsules.

Another lady, who started to take the deep sea shark liver oil capsules daily as a prophylactic against the regular development of cold sores in wintertime, had an interesting story to tell me because it concerned a cosmetic influence of the product. Cold sores are caused by the Herpes simplex virus. There are two types of this Herpes simplex virus, and it is mainly Herpes type 1 that causes cold sores, although type 2 can be involved. Because it is a viral disease, the most effective treatments work through internal immune reactions, and thus immunostimulatory products such as deep sea shark liver oil can help reduce the symptoms.

The lady related that after a few weeks of taking the capsules on a regular daily basis she noticed that her general skin condition had improved significantly. The improvement she described was that her skin felt smoother and silkier. Also, she felt that her face looked fresher and possibly even a bit younger. She was very pleased with this secondary effect and had reduced her use of facial cosmetics.

I can imagine the skeptical reader thinking that the fresher-faced, younger look was probably wishful thinking! However, having met the lady in question I can vouch for the fact that she certainly looked fresh-faced, healthy, and younger than her age. How could this be? First, I think we would all agree that a fresh, healthy skin normally gives a younger appearance than an unhealthy skin. Second, we should remember that the deep sea shark liver oil contains between 35 and 40 percent squalene. As we have seen earlier in the book, squalene is noted for its emollient, antioxidant, and healthy skin properties—hence its use by the cosmetic industry.

These anecdotes are just a few of the experiences related by people who, usually because of recommendation by a friend or relative, but sometimes because nothing else has seemed to help, have tried these particular products of the seas. They represent some of the success stories, of which there are many. Of course there have also been stories of disappointment because the products did not help. This is quite normal since no product has a 100 percent success rate. There will always be some who benefit and some who do not from the same treatment. For those who do not benefit from these products, I hope that they are able to find a treatment from another source that can provide similar benefit and lack of adverse side effects. For the many who may benefit, I hope that this book, and in particular this chapter, might just provide the inspiration to try these products from the seas.

REFERENCES

CHAPTER 2

Harada, H. et al. Oral taurine supplementation prevents the development of ethanol-induced hypertension in rats. *Hypertens Res* 23(3): 277–284, 2000.

CHAPTER 3

Ankenbauer-Perkins, K.; Slacek, B.; Alexander, A.; Pollard, B.; Guilford, G.; Marshal, A.; and Hedderley, D. The efficacy of Green-Lipped Mussel Extract in the management of degenerative joint disease in dogs. Awaiting publication.

Audeval, B. and Bouchacourt, P. Double-blind, placebo-controlled study of the mussel *Perna canaliculus* (New Zealand green-lipped mussel) in gonarthrosis (arthritis of the knee). *La Gazette Medicale*, 93(38):111–115, 1986.

Caughey, D. E.; Grigor, R. R.; Caughey, E. B.; Young, P.; Gow, P. J.; and Stewart, A. W. *Perna canaliculus* in the treatment of rheumatoid arthritis. *J Rheumatoidal Inflammation*, 6:197–200, 1983.

Couch, R. A. F.; Ormrod, D. J.; Miller, T. E.; and Watkins, W. B. Anti-inflammatory activity in fractionated extracts of the green-lipped mussel. *NZ Med J*, 720:803–6, 1982.

Davis, P. F. et al. Inhibition of angiogenesis by oral ingestion of shark cartilage in a rat model. *Microvascular Research*, 54:178–182, 1997.

Gibson, R. G.; Gibson, S. L. M.; Conway, V. et al. *Perna canaliculus* in the treatment of arthritis. *Practitioner*, 224:955–60, 1980.

Hawkins T. The effects of chiropractic mobilisation and oral administration of Seatone in the treatment of osteoarthritis of the knee joint. Thesis submitted to Faculty of Health Sciences, Technicon Witwatersrand, South Africa, 2001.

Hazelton, R. A. Adapted from Promotional Literature. C-cure in rheumatoid arthritis: a six-month placebo-controlled study. University of Queensland, Australia, 1995.

Huskisson, E. C.; Scot, J.; and Bryans, R. Short Reports, Seatone is ineffective in rheumatoid arthritis. *BMJ*, 281:1358, 1981.

Kendall, R.; Lawson, J.; and Hurley, L. A. New research and a clinical report on the use of *Perna canaliculus* in the management of arthritis. *Townsend Letter for Doctors and Patients*, 204:98–111, 2000.

Knaus, U. G.; Tubar, A.; and Wagner, H. Pharmacological properties of glycogens: anti-complementary and anti-inflammatory action of mussel glycogen (*Perna canaliculus*). Dept of Immunology Imm2, Scripps Clinic and Research Foundation, La Jolla, California, USA. Also Universities of Trieste, Italy, and Munich, Germany, 1990.

Kosuge, T.; Tsuji, K.; Ishida, H.; and Yamaguchi, T. Isolation of an anti-histaminic substance from green-lipped mussel (*Perna canaliculus*). *Chem Pharm Bull*, 34:4825–8, 1986.

Lambert, M. et al. The ergogenic properties of New Zealand Green-Lipped Mussel Extract. Research report by MRC/UCT Bioenergetics of Exercise Research Unit, UCT Medical School, Sports Science Institute of South Africa; 1998.

Lambert, M.; Semark, A.; and Grobler, L. The ergogenic properties of Seatone. Awaiting publication.

Larkin, J. G.; Capell, H. A.; and Sturrock, R. D. Seatone in rheumatoid arthritis: a six-month placebo-controlled study. *Annals of Rheumatic Diseases*, 44:199–201, 1985.

Miller, T. E. and Ormrod, D. J. The anti-inflammatory activity of *Perna canaliculus* (New Zealand Green-Lipped Mussel). *NZ Med J*, 667: 187–193, 1980.

Miller, T. E. and Wu, H. In vivo evidence for prostaglandin inhibitory activity in New Zealand Green-Lipped Mussel Extract. *NZ Med J*, 97:355–7, 1984.

Miller, T. E. et al. Relationship between suppression of neutrophil function and increase in infection. Adapted from paper in *Brit J Exp Path*, 67:13–23, 1986.

Miller, T. E.; Dodd, J.; Ormrod, D. J.; and Geddes, R. Anti-inflammatory activity of glycogen extracted from *Perna canaliculus* (NZ green-lipped mussel). *Agents and Actions*, 38:Special Conference Issue, 1993.

Miller, T. E.; Ormrod, D. J.; and Findon, G. Evaluation of the effect of Seatone administration on cell-mediated immune mechanisms determined using "in vitro" and "in vivo" analysis of T lymphocyte function. Private study in the Department of Medicine, University of Auckland, 1984.

Oikawa, T. et al. A novel angiogenic inhibitor derived from Japanese shark cartilage. Extraction and estimation of inhibitory activities toward tumour and embryonic angiogenesis. *Cancer Lett*, 51:181–186, 1990.

Orima, H.; Fujita, M.; Omura, T.; and Kirihara, N. Clinical effects of the extract of the New Zealand green-lipped mussel on dogs and cats with joint diseases. Private study conducted by the Nippon Veterinary and Animal Science University, Japan, 1998.

Rainsford, K. D. and Whitehouse, M. W. Gastroprotective and anti-inflammatory properties of green-lipped mussel (*Perna canaliculus*) preparation. *Drug Res*, 12(11):30, 1980.

Whitehouse, M. W. et al. Anti-inflammatory activity of a Holothurian (sea cucumber) food supplement in rats. *Inflammopharmacology*, 2: 411–417, 1994.

Yaacob, H. B. et al. Antinociceptive effect of the water extract of Malaysian sea cucumber. *Asia Pacific Journal of Pharmacology*, 9:23–28, 1994.

CHAPTER 4

Ormrod, D. J. et al. Dietary chitosan inhibits hypercholesterolaemia and atherogenesis in the apolipoprotein E-deficient mouse model of atherosclerosis. *Atherosclerosis*, 138:329–334, 1998.

Maezaki, Y. et al. Hypocholesterolemic effect of chitosan in adult males. *Biosci Biotech Biochem*, 57(9):1439–1444, 1993.

CHAPTER 5

Andreesen, R. et al. Selective destruction of human leukemic cells by alkyllysophospholipids. *Cancer Res*, 38:3894, 1978.

Berdel, W. E. et al. The influence of alkylphospholipids and lysophospholipids activated macrophages on the development of metastasis of Lewis lung carcinoma. *Eur J Cancer*, 16:1199, 1980.

Boeryd, B. et al. Stimulation of immune reactivity by methoxy-substituted glycerol ethers incorporated into the feed. *Eur J Immunol*, 8:678–680, 1978.

Brohult, A. et al. Effect of alkoxyglycerols on the frequency of injuries following radiation therapy for carcinoma of the uterine cervix. *Acta Obstet Gynecol Scand*, 56:441–448, 1977.

D'Amore, P. A. Antiangiogenesis as a strategy for antimetastasis. *Seminars in Thrombosis and Hemostasis*, 14(1):73–78, 1988.

Lane, I. W. et al. *Sharks Don't Get Cancer: How Shark Cartilage Could Save Your Life*. New York: Avery, 1992.

Lane, I. W. et al. *Sharks Still Don't Get Cancer*. New York: Avery, 1996.

Modelell, M. et al. Disturbance of phospholipid metabolism during selective destruction of tumour cells induced by alkylphospholipids. *Cancer Res*, 38:4681, 1979.

Pugliese, P. T. et al. Some biological actions of alkylglycerols from shark liver oil. *The Journal of Alternative and Complementary Medicine*, 4:87–99, 1998.

Wagner, B. A. et al. Membrane peroxidative damage enhancement by the ether lipids class of antineoplastic agents. *Cancer Res*, 52:6045–6057, 1992.

Weidner, N. et al. Tumor angiogenesis and metastasis—correlation in invasive breast carcinoma. *The New England Journal of Medicine*, 324(1): 1–8, 1991.

Yamamoto, N. et al. Activation of mouse macrophages by alkylglycerols, inflammation products of cancerous tissues. *Cancer Res*, 48:6044–6049, 1998.

CHAPTER 6

Boeryd, B. et al. Stimulation of immune reactivity by methoxy-substituted glycerol ethers incorporated into the feed. *Eur J Immunol*, 8:678–680, 1978.

Wagner, B. A. et al. Membrane peroxidative damage enhancement by the ether lipids class of antineoplastic agents. *Cancer Res*, 52:6045–6057, 1992.

Yamamoto, N. et al. Activation of mouse macrophages by alkylglycerols, inflammation products of cancerous tissues. *Cancer Res*, 48:6044–6049, 1998.

CHAPTER 8

Maezaki, Y. et al. Hypocholesterolemic effect of chitosan in adult males. *Biosci Biotech Biochem*, 57(9):1439–1444, 1993.

Nauss, J. L. et al. The binding of micellar lipids to chitosan. *Lipids*, 18: 714–719, 1983.

CHAPTER 9

Banderet, L. E. Treatment with tyrosine a neurotransmitter precursor, reduces environmental stress in humans. *Brain Res Bull*, 22:759–762, 1989.

Braverman, E. R. *The Healing Nutrients Within.* New Canaan, Connecticut, USA: Keats Publishing, 1997, pp. 58–59.

Brown, D. et al. Natural remedies for depression. *Nutrition Science News*, February 1999.

Cangiono, C. et al. Eating behaviour and adherence to dietary prescriptions in obese subjects treated with 5-hydroxytryptophan. *American Journal of Clinical Nutrition*, 56:863–868, 1992.

Deijen, J. B. et al. Effect of tyrosine on cognitive function and blood pressure under stress. *Brain Res Bull*, 33(3):319–323, 1994.

Den Boer, J. A. et al. Behavioural neuroendocrine and biochemical effects of 5-hydroxytryptophan administration in panic disorder. *Psychiatry Research*, 31:262–278, 1990.

Erdmann, R. et al. *The Amino Revolution.* London, UK: Century Hutchinson, 1987, pp. 66–67.

Gelenberd, A. J. et al. Tyrosine for the treatment of depression. *American Journal of Psychiatry*, 137:622–623, 1980.

Kahn, R. S. et al. L-5-hydroxytryptophan in the treatment of anxiety disorder. *Journal of Affective Disorders*, 8:197–200, 1995.

Mai, C. A. et al. Dietary tyrosine as an aid to stress resistance among troops. *Military Medicine*, 154(3):144, 1989.

Reinstein, D. K. et al. Dietary tyrosine suppresses the rise in plasma corticosterone following acute stress in rats. *Life Sciences*, 37:2157–2163, 1985.

Sourlairac, A. et al. Action of 5-hydroxytryptophan, serotonin precursor, on insomniacs. *Annals Medicon Psychologiques*, 135:792–798, 1977.

Van Hiel, L. J. L-5-hydroxytryptophan in depression: the first substitution therapy in psychiatry? The treatment of 99 outpatients with "therapy-resistant" depression. *Neuropsychobiology*, 6:230–240, 1980.

CHAPTER 11

Clark, L. Chapter 8 of *Are You Radioactive?*. Greenwich, CT: Devin-Adair, 1974.

Tanaka et al. Studies on inhibition of intestinal absorption of radioactive strontium (Sea Vegetables). *Canadian Medical Journal*, 99:169–75, 1968.

INDEX

Fibrositis, *see lumbago*
Fluoride, 3, 87–88
Free radicals, 32–33, 77, 78

Glucosamines, 29
Glycerol, 54
Glycosaminoglycans, *see
mucopolysaccharides*
Goiter, 85, 86–88
Gout, 31

Halichondrin B, 4
Heart disease, 37–40, 63–70
Hepatitis (A or B), 49
Herpes simplex, 116–117
High blood pressure, 37, 63
High-density lipoprotein, 65, 69
Homeostasis, 14
Hypercholesterolemia, 39
Hyperlipidemia, 63–70
Hyperthyroidism, 87
Hypoglycemia, 8
Hypothyroidism, 87

Immune system, 49–56, 60
Immunity
    acquired, 51
    active, 52
    artificial, 52
    natural, 51
    passive, 52
Immunomodulation, 60
Influenza, 49, 114–115
Iodine, 3, 86, 88

Kelp, 86, 88, 92

Laulimalide, 4
Leucocytes, 50, 53
Leukemias, 41, 42
Leukotrienes, 16, 28, 30, 59
Lipids, 38, 39, 64, 65, 69
Liver damage, 8, 11
Lockjaw, *see tetanus*
Low-density lipoprotein, 65, 69
Lumbago (Fibrositis), 16
Lymph, 50

Lymphocytes, 42, 50–51, 55
Lymphomas, 41, 42

Macrophages, 45, 46, 54–55
Magnesium, 8, 10–11
Marine farming, 5–6, 89–99
    abalone, 93–94
    aesthetic impact of, 98
    cod, 90
    environmental factors in,
        94–99
    mussels, 89, 91–92
    navigational impacts of, 98
    oysters, 91, 93
    seahorses, 94
    seaweeds, 92
    sponges, 92–93
    starfish, 92
Measles, 51
Melanomas, 41
Mental acuity, 72, 76, 77–80
Mental health, 71–80
Mineral depletion, 8, 10, 11
Mucopolysaccharides
    (glycosaminoglycans),
    29–30, 31, 32, 34

National Cancer Institute, 3, 43
Neutrophils, 27, 28, 30, 35, 55
New Zealand green-lipped
    mussel, 21, 89
    extract of, 21–31, 34, 35,
        102–114
Norepinephrine, 75

Omega-3 fatty acids, 65–67, 79,
    80
Omega-6 fatty acids, 79, 80
Osteoarthritis, 13, 14, 15, 34
Osteoporosis, 8, 29, 81–84
Oxidative burst, 55
Oyster
    extract, 9, 11
    shell, 83

Panic disorder, 74
Plaque, 37, 38, 65, 66

Saxtles' dogfish.

Poliomyelitis, 52
Polyculture, 93
Prostaglandins, 16, 28, 30, 66
Proteoglycan, 30
Psoriasis, 57, 58–59

Radiation
    sickness, 85–86
    therapy, 42, 44, 45, 46
Rheumatoid Arthritis, 15–16, 17,
    31
Rickets, 83
Rubella, *see measles*

Scarlet fever, 51
Sea cucumber, 34–35
Sea urchin, 34
Seawater
    as antibiotic, 2
    mineral composition of, 3
Seaweed, 4, 86
Serotonin, 74, 75
Sexual dysfunction, 8
Shark cartilage, 31–33, 34, 46
Shark liver oil, 43–46, 53–56, 60,
    114–117
Skin diseases, *see dermatological
    diseases*
Sponges, marine, 3, 4, 43
Squalene, 61, 80
Squid pen, 38
Starfish, 4, 34
Statins, 38
Still's disease, 17

Stress, 18–21, 71–72
Symbiosis, 93

Taurine, 9–11
Tennis elbow, 17
Tetanus (Lockjaw), 52, 53
Tetrodotoxin, 1
Thromboxanes, 66
Thymus, 50
Thyroid gland, 85, 86–88
Triglycerides, 66, 67
Tryptophan, 74, 75, 76
Tuberculosis, 52
Tumors, 41, 45, 46, 47
Tyrosine, 75–76

Urinary incontinence, 94

Viral disorders, 49–56, 60, 114,
    116–117
Vitamin
    A, 56, 60
    B12, 10, 11
    B group, 8, 10, 88
    D, 56, 60, 83
    E, 60
Vitamin depletion, 8, 10, 11

White blood cells, 42, 44, 50, 53,
    54, 55
Whooping cough, 52

Zinc, 3, 8, 10–11

MORE TITLES
FROM VITAL HEALTH PUBLISHING:

Trace Your Genes to Health, Chris Reading, M.D., with Ross Meillon, 336 pages, 1-890612-23-5, $15.95.

Our Children's Health: America's Kids in Nutritional Crisis & How We Can Help, Bonnie Minsky, M.A., C.N.S., M.P.H., Lisa Holk, N.D. 296 pages, 1-890612-27-8, $15.95.

Smart Nutrients (new 2nd ed.), Abram Hoffer, M.D., Ph.D., Morton Walker, D.P.M., 224 pages, 1-890612-26-X, $14.95.

Stevia Sweet Recipes: Sugar-Free–Naturally! (2nd ed.), Jeffrey Goettemoeller, 200 pages, 1-890612-13-8, $13.95.

The Asthma Breakthrough: Breathe Freely–Naturally! Henry Osiecki, B.Sc., 192 pages, 1-890612-22-7, $13.95.

Nutrition in a Nutshell: Build Health and Slow Down the Aging Process, Bonnie Minsky, L.C.N., M.A., 196 pages, 1-890612-17-0, $14.95.

Wheatgrass: Superfood for a New Millenium, Li Smith, 164 pages, 1-890612-10-3, $10.95.

Energy For Life: How to Overcome Chronic Fatigue, George Redmon, Ph.D., N.D., approx. 240 pages, 1-890612-14-6, $15.95.

The Cancer Handbook: What's Really Working, edited by Lynne McTaggart, 192 pages, 1-890612-18-9, $12.95.

Taste Life! The Organic Choice, Ed. by David Richard and Dorie Byers, R.N., 208 pages, 1-890612-08-1, $12.95.

Healthy Living: A Holistic Guide to Cleansing, Revitalization and Nutrition, Susana Lombard, 112 pages, 1-890612-30-8, $12.95.

Stevia Rebaudiana: Nature's Sweet Secret, (3rd ed.) David Richard, 80 pages, 1-890612-15-4, $7.95. Includes growing info.

Healing Herb Rapid Reference, Brent Davis, D.C., 148 pages, 1-890612-21-9, $12.95.

Natural Beauty Basics: Create Your Own Cosmetics and Body Care Products, Dorie Byers, R.N., 208 pages, 1-890612-19-7, $14.95.

OTHER TITLES
FROM ENHANCEMENT BOOKS:

Facets of a Diamond, Reflections of a Healer, John Diamond, M.D., 336 pages, 1-890995-17-7, $16.95.

The Veneration of Life: Through the Disease to the Soul, John Diamond, M.D., 80 pages, 1-890995-14-2, $9.95.

The Way of the Pulse: Drumming With Spirit, John Diamond, M.D., 116 pages, 1-890995-02-9, $13.95.

The Healing Power of Blake: A Distillation, edited by John Diamond, M.D., 180 pages, 1-890995-03-7, $14.95.

The Healer: Heart and Hearth, John Diamond, M.D., 112 pages, 1-890995-22-3, $13.95.

Holism and Beyond: The Essence of Holistic Medicine, John Diamond, M.D., 48 pages, 1-890995-17-7, $8.95.

Music and Song, Mother and Love, John Diamond, M.D., 136 pages, 1-890995-33-9, $13.95.

Every Breath You Take: Revolutionary Asthma Treatment, Paul J. Ameisen, N.D., 200 pages, 1-890995-47-9, $10.95.

Life Enhancement Through Music, John Diamond, M.D., approx. 176 pages, 1-890995-01-0, $14.95.

I Love What I Do! A Drummer's Philosophy of Life at Eighty, Sam Ulano, 168 pages, 1-890995-35-5, $14.95.

Someone Hurt Me, Susan Cavaciuti, 48 pages, color illustrated, children's, 1-890995-20-7, $8.95.

Enhancement Books
P.O. Box 152
Ridgefield, CT 06877
www.vitalhealth.net
info@vitalhealth.net
877-VIT-BOOK

RESOURCES

For further information on the marine products described in this book, please contact:

INTERNATIONALLY:

J. E. Croft
174, Foley Quarry Road, RD 2
Albany, Aukland, New Zealand
EMAIL: scimar@xtra.co.nz

Healtheries of New Zealand Ltd.
PO Box 22 045
Otahuhu, Auckland, New Zealand
EMAIL : webmail@healtheries.co.nz

WITHIN THE USA:

Marine Nutriceutical Corporation
794 Sunrise Boulevard
Mt. Bethel, PA 18343
PHONE: 570-897-0351
TOLL FREE: 866-627-4631
FAX: 570-897-7732
WEBSITE: www.marine-ingredients.com